# PERIPHERAL NEUROPATHY DIET COOKBOOK FOR BEGINNERS

Delicious, Easy-to-Follow Recipes to Soothe Nerve Pain, Reduce Inflammation, and Enhance Overall Well-being

Kingsley Klopp

**To show our appreciation for your purchase, we're delighted to offer you these special bonuses as a heartfelt thank you**

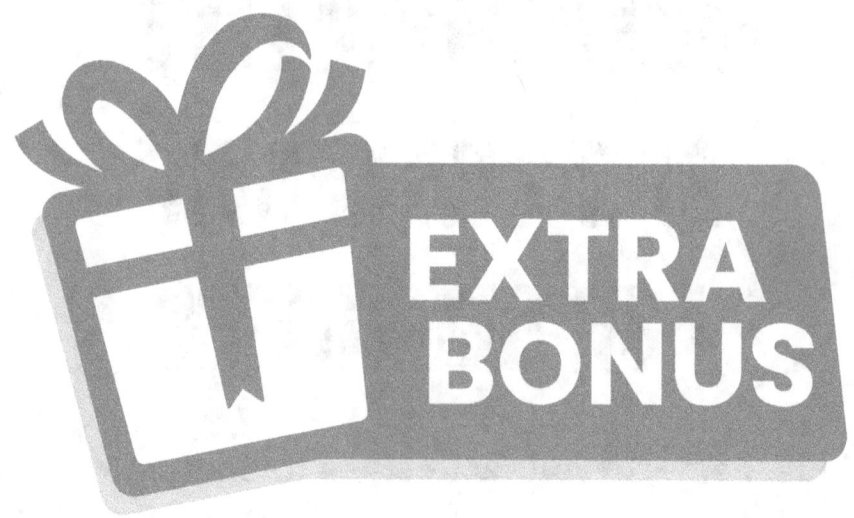

1. A Food Tracker Journal
2. Downloadable E-BOOK featuring full-color images of finished recipes

**Copyright © 2024 All rights reserved.**

No part of this book may be reproduced or transmitted in any form or by any means, electronic or mechanical, including photocopying, recording, or by any information storage and retrieval system, without written permission from the author. The scanning, uploading, and distribution of this book via the internet or via any other means without the permission of the author is illegal and punishable by law. The author has made every effort to ensure the accuracy of the information contained in this book. However, the author cannot be held responsible for any errors or omissions.

# Table of Contents

Introduction..........................................................................................................7

## Part 1
**Understanding Peripheral Neuropathy**
- What is Peripheral Neuropathy?................................................................9
- Common Causes and Symptoms..............................................................11
- How Diet Can Influence Neuropathy........................................................13

## Part 2
**The Role of Diet in Managing Peripheral Neuropathy**
- Key Nutrients for Nerve Health..................................................................15
- Foods to Avoid..............................................................................................18

**Breakfast Recipes**
Avocado Toast with Poached Egg.................................................................20
Quinoa Porridge...............................................................................................21
Oatmeal with Mixed Berries..........................................................................22
Smoothie Bowl.................................................................................................23
Vegetable Omelet............................................................................................24
Banana Pancakes............................................................................................25
Sweet Potato Hash..........................................................................................26
Nutty Rice Pudding.........................................................................................27
Buckwheat Crepes..........................................................................................28
Muesli and Yogurt............................................................................................29
Spinach and Feta Wrap..................................................................................30
Almond Butter and Banana Sandwich.........................................................31
Egg Muffins.......................................................................................................32
Tofu Scramble..................................................................................................33
Pumpkin Oatmeal............................................................................................34
Turkey Sausage and Veggie Skillet...............................................................35
Ricotta and Tomato Toast..............................................................................36

Breakfast Lentils...........................................................................................................37
Mango and Coconut Rice...........................................................................................38
Savory Porridge...........................................................................................................39
Stuffed Breakfast Peppers..........................................................................................40
Apple-Cinnamon Oat Bake.........................................................................................41
Almond Flour Waffles.................................................................................................42
Zucchini and Onion Frittata.......................................................................................43
Shakshuka....................................................................................................................44

## Fish and Seafood Recipes
Grilled Salmon with Dill Yogurt Sauce......................................................................45
Baked Cod with Lemon and Capers..........................................................................46
Shrimp and Avocado Salad.........................................................................................47
Herb-Crusted Tilapia...................................................................................................48
Scallop Stir-Fry.............................................................................................................49
Fish Tacos with Cabbage Slaw....................................................................................50
Crab Stuffed Mushrooms............................................................................................51
Tuna Nicoise Salad.......................................................................................................52
Lemon Garlic Shrimp...................................................................................................53
Mackerel Pate................................................................................................................54
Baked Trout with Almonds.........................................................................................55
Haddock in Parchment................................................................................................56
Scallop and Pea Risotto...............................................................................................57
Grilled Tuna Steaks......................................................................................................58
Sardines on Toast.........................................................................................................59
Mussels in Tomato Broth............................................................................................60
Ceviche..........................................................................................................................61
Sea Bass with Mango Salsa.........................................................................................62
Garlic Butter Scallops..................................................................................................63
Parmesan Crusted Halibut.........................................................................................64
Spicy Tuna Roll............................................................................................................65
Fish Curry.....................................................................................................................66
Grilled Shrimp and Vegetable Bowl..........................................................................67
Salmon and Spinach Quiche......................................................................................68
Kedgeree.......................................................................................................................69
Seafood Fettuccine......................................................................................................70

## Vegetables
Roasted Brussels Sprouts with Balsamic Glaze........................................................71
Spiced Sweet Potato Soup..........................................................................................72
Kale and Quinoa Salad................................................................................................73
Grilled Vegetable Platter.............................................................................................74

Carrot and Coriander Soup...................................................................................75
Zucchini Noodles with Pesto..................................................................................76
Cauliflower Steaks with Herb Sauce.......................................................................77
Eggplant Parmesan...............................................................................................78
Spaghetti Squash with Tomato Sauce....................................................................79
Butternut Squash Risotto.......................................................................................80
Curried Lentils with Spinach..................................................................................81
Mushroom Stroganoff............................................................................................82
Garlic Green Beans................................................................................................83
Vegetable Stir-Fry with Tofu..................................................................................84
Tomato Gazpacho.................................................................................................85
Cabbage Slaw with Sesame Dressing....................................................................86
Roasted Turnips with Rosemary............................................................................87
Sautéed Swiss Chard with Pine Nuts.....................................................................88
Vegan Ratatouille..................................................................................................89
 Spinach and Feta Pie............................................................................................90
Pumpkin Chili........................................................................................................91
Grilled Asparagus with Lemon Tarragon Dressing.................................................92
Vegetable Paella....................................................................................................93
Mashed Cauliflower with Chives............................................................................94
Roasted Radishes with Soy Sauce.........................................................................95

**Poultry Recipes**
Grilled Chicken with Avocado Salsa.......................................................................96
Turkey and Spinach Meatballs...............................................................................97
 Lemon Herb Roasted Chicken..............................................................................98
Chicken Stir-Fry with Broccoli................................................................................99
Baked Pesto Chicken...........................................................................................100
Smoked Paprika Chicken.....................................................................................101
Asian Turkey Lettuce Wraps................................................................................102
Chicken and Asparagus Skillet.............................................................................103
Turkey Stuffed Peppers.......................................................................................104
Buffalo Chicken Salad..........................................................................................105
Chicken Cacciatore..............................................................................................106
Turkey Burgers with Sweet Potato Fries..............................................................107
Chicken and Mushroom Risotto...........................................................................108
Grilled Turkey Kebabs.........................................................................................109
Slow Cooker Chicken Tikka Masala.....................................................................110
Greek Chicken Bowls...........................................................................................111
 Honey Mustard Chicken Thighs.........................................................................112
Pulled Turkey Tacos............................................................................................113
Balsamic Chicken and Vegetables.......................................................................114

Barbecue Chicken Pizza...............................................................................................115
Turkey Sloppy Joes........................................................................................................116
Chicken and Spinach Stuffed Shells..........................................................................117
Lemon Garlic Turkey Breast........................................................................................118
Chicken Paillard.............................................................................................................119
 Turkey Meatloaf............................................................................................................120

**10-WEEK MEAL PLAN**..............................................................................................121

## Important Note

We're thrilled to have you join us on this journey towards better health and well-being through the power of nutrition. As you explore these pages, filled with delicious and nutritious recipes designed to support your nerve health, we want to share a few important reminders to ensure you get the most out of this culinary adventure.

Each of us is unique, and our bodies have different needs. What works wonders for one person might not be as effective for another. Peripheral neuropathy can manifest in various ways, and dietary responses can vary widely. We encourage you to listen to your body and adjust the recipes to meet your personal needs and preferences. Feel free to experiment and modify ingredients to suit your tastes and health goals. If you have any dietary restrictions or specific health concerns, it's always a good idea to tailor the recipes accordingly.

Navigating a new diet, especially one aimed at managing a health condition like peripheral neuropathy, can sometimes be confusing or overwhelming. If you ever feel unsure about a particular ingredient or dietary change, we strongly recommend consulting with your healthcare provider. Your doctor can provide personalized advice based on your medical history and current health status, ensuring that your dietary choices are safe and beneficial.

We've provided nutritional information for each recipe to help you make informed decisions about your meals. However, it's important to note that these values are approximate and can vary based on the specific ingredients and brands you use. Factors such as portion sizes, cooking methods, and ingredient variations can all influence the nutritional content. We encourage you to use this information as a general guide rather than an exact measurement.

Furthermore, If our cookbook has brought joy to your kitchen and table, we'd be thrilled to hear about your experiences in an Amazon review. On the flip side, if you stumble upon any hiccups while exploring our recipes, don't hesitate to get in touch at **kloppkingsley@gmail.com.** We're here to support your cooking journey every step of the way.

# Introduction

Welcome to the *Peripheral Neuropathy Diet Cookbook for Beginners*! If you're here, it's likely that you or someone you care about is dealing with the challenges of peripheral neuropathy. This condition, which affects the nerves outside the brain and spinal cord, can cause a host of debilitating symptoms such as pain, tingling, numbness, and muscle weakness. Living with these symptoms can be incredibly tough, but the good news is that you've taken a proactive step towards managing your condition through diet. This cookbook is designed to be your guide, your companion, and your support system on this journey. Imagine waking up each day with less discomfort, more energy, and a renewed sense of hope. Picture yourself enjoying meals that are not only delicious but also tailored to help reduce your symptoms and improve your overall well-being. This is not just a cookbook; it's a blueprint for a healthier, more comfortable life. The recipes and meal plans within these pages are crafted to support your nerve health, reduce inflammation, and provide the essential nutrients your body needs to combat peripheral neuropathy. But let's start with a bit of a reality check. We know that changing your diet isn't always easy. It requires commitment, perseverance, and a willingness to try new things. You might be wondering if you have the time, the skills, or the energy to make such a change. The answer is: Yes, you do. And we're here to help you every step of the way. Whether you're a seasoned cook or someone who is just starting to find their way around the kitchen, this cookbook is designed with you in mind. We've included simple, easy-to-follow recipes that are both nutritious and delicious, ensuring that you won't feel deprived or overwhelmed.

Why is diet so important for managing peripheral neuropathy? The foods we eat play a crucial role in our body's ability to heal and function properly. Certain foods can exacerbate inflammation and worsen your symptoms, while others can help to soothe and repair nerve damage. This cookbook is packed with recipes that include anti-inflammatory ingredients, rich in vitamins and minerals that are essential for nerve health. Think of your meals as medicine – each bite is a step towards reducing your pain and improving your quality of life. Let's talk about some of the stars of your new diet. Leafy greens, lean proteins, whole grains, nuts, seeds, and a rainbow of fruits and vegetables will become your best friends. These foods are packed with antioxidants, healthy fats, and essential nutrients like B vitamins, which are vital for nerve function. You'll also find recipes that exclude common culprits that can aggravate neuropathy, such as excessive sugar, refined grains, and unhealthy fats. But don't worry – you won't miss out on flavor. Our recipes are designed to be satisfying and delicious, proving that healthy eating can be a pleasure, not a chore.

In addition to the recipes, we've included meal plans and shopping lists to make your transition as smooth as possible. We understand that life is busy, and finding time to plan meals can be a challenge. Our goal is to take the guesswork out of your meal preparation, so you can focus on what's most important – your health and well-being. We also encourage you to track your progress and listen to your body. Everyone's experience with peripheral neuropathy is unique, and what works for one person might not work for another. By paying attention to how different foods affect your symptoms, you can fine-tune your diet to best suit your needs.

So, are you ready to embark on this journey towards better health? With this cookbook in hand, you have the tools, the knowledge, and the support to make a real difference in your life. Here's to flavorful meals, reduced symptoms, and a brighter, healthier future. Let's get cooking!

# Part 1

# Understanding Peripheral Neuropathy

## *What is Peripheral Neuropathy?*

Peripheral neuropathy is a condition that affects the peripheral nerves, which are the nerves outside of the brain and spinal cord. These nerves play a crucial role in connecting the central nervous system to the rest of the body, enabling sensations and movements. When these nerves are damaged, it can lead to a wide array of distressing and often debilitating symptoms that impact every aspect of daily life. Imagine waking up one day and feeling a strange tingling in your feet, a sensation that refuses to go away. Over time, this tingling evolves into a persistent numbness and then, more alarmingly, into sharp, burning pain that travels up your legs. The simple act of walking, which you once took for granted, becomes a painful ordeal. This is the harsh reality faced by those with peripheral neuropathy. Peripheral neuropathy can affect sensory nerves, motor nerves, or autonomic nerves. Sensory nerves control the sensations of touch, temperature, and pain. When these nerves are damaged, it can result in unusual and painful sensations, such as tingling, numbness, and burning. Motor nerves control muscle movements, and damage to these nerves can lead to muscle weakness, loss of coordination, and even paralysis. Autonomic nerves regulate involuntary functions like heart rate, blood pressure, and digestion. Damage to these nerves can cause symptoms like dizziness, bladder problems, and digestive issues.

Living with peripheral neuropathy is often an emotional and physical roller coaster. The pain and discomfort can be relentless, affecting not only the person suffering but also their loved ones. There is a sense of loss that accompanies this condition—the loss of independence, the loss of mobility, and the loss of comfort in one's own body. Each step can be a reminder of the condition's presence, making every day a challenge. What makes peripheral neuropathy particularly heart-wrenching is its unpredictability. The symptoms can vary widely from person to person and can change in intensity and nature over time. For some, the symptoms might be mild and manageable, while for others, they can be severe and life-altering. This unpredictability can lead to feelings of anxiety and helplessness, as it's difficult to know what each day will bring.

One of the most challenging aspects of peripheral neuropathy is the impact it has on mental health. Chronic pain and discomfort can lead to depression, anxiety, and a sense of isolation. The constant battle with pain can be exhausting, both physically and emotionally. Many people with peripheral neuropathy find themselves withdrawing from social activities and the things they once loved, further contributing to their sense of isolation and despair. However, amidst the pain and struggle, there is also a story of resilience and hope. Many individuals with peripheral neuropathy find ways to adapt and manage their condition, discovering new strategies and treatments that help them reclaim their lives. This journey often requires a great deal of courage and perseverance, as it involves navigating a complex landscape of medical treatments, lifestyle changes, and emotional challenges.

Support from loved ones and healthcare professionals is crucial in this journey. Empathy and understanding from those around can make a significant difference, offering a lifeline of support and comfort. It's important for those suffering to know they are not alone and that their pain is acknowledged and validated. In the face of peripheral neuropathy, hope can be found in small victories—moments of reduced pain, a good night's sleep, the ability to walk a bit further than yesterday. These victories are a testament to the strength and resilience of those living with this condition. They serve as reminders that while peripheral neuropathy can be a formidable adversary, it does not define the entirety of a person's life.

# Common Causes and Symptoms of Peripheral Neuropathy

## Common Causes

1. Diabetes: One of the most prevalent causes of peripheral neuropathy is diabetes. High blood sugar levels over time can damage nerves throughout the body, leading to diabetic neuropathy. This condition often affects the legs and feet first, causing pain, tingling, and loss of sensation.
2. Alcoholism: Chronic alcohol consumption can lead to nutritional deficiencies, particularly of vitamins B1, B6, B12, and folate, which are essential for nerve health. Alcohol also has a direct toxic effect on peripheral nerves, resulting in alcoholic neuropathy.
3. Autoimmune Diseases: Conditions such as rheumatoid arthritis, lupus, and Guillain-Barré syndrome can cause the body's immune system to attack its own nerves. This autoimmune response can result in significant nerve damage and subsequent neuropathy.
4. Infections: Certain infections can lead to peripheral neuropathy. These include Lyme disease, shingles (herpes zoster), HIV/AIDS, and hepatitis C. The infection can directly damage nerves or cause inflammation that leads to neuropathy.
5. Inherited Disorders: Some types of peripheral neuropathy are hereditary. Charcot-Marie-Tooth disease is one of the most common inherited neurological disorders, affecting the peripheral nerves and leading to muscle weakness and sensory loss.
6. Trauma or Nerve Injury: Physical injury from accidents, falls, or surgeries can damage peripheral nerves. Repetitive stress injuries, such as carpal tunnel syndrome, can also compress and damage nerves, leading to neuropathy.
7. Exposure to Toxins: Certain chemicals and toxins, including heavy metals like lead and mercury, can cause nerve damage. Exposure to industrial chemicals, pesticides, and some medications, such as chemotherapy drugs, can also result in peripheral neuropathy.
8. Kidney and Liver Disorders: When the kidneys or liver fail to function properly, toxins build up in the blood, which can damage nerves. Chronic kidney disease and liver cirrhosis are notable conditions that can lead to neuropathy.
9. Vitamin Deficiencies: Deficiencies in vitamins essential for nerve health, such as B vitamins, vitamin E, and niacin, can lead to neuropathy. Poor diet, malabsorption disorders, and certain medical conditions can contribute to these deficiencies.
10. Cancer and Chemotherapy: Both cancer itself and its treatments can cause peripheral neuropathy. Some cancers, particularly those involving the blood or bone marrow, can affect nerve function. Chemotherapy-induced peripheral neuropathy (CIPN) is a common side effect of cancer treatment.

## Common Symptoms

The symptoms of peripheral neuropathy can vary greatly depending on the type of nerves affected—sensory, motor, or autonomic—and the severity of the damage. Here are some of the most common symptoms:

1. Sensory Symptoms:
   - Numbness and Tingling: Often starting in the hands and feet, these sensations can spread up the limbs. The feeling is akin to "pins and needles" and can be persistent or intermittent.
   - Burning Pain: Many individuals with neuropathy describe a burning or shooting pain, which can be severe and debilitating. This pain often worsens at night, affecting sleep.
   - Sensitivity to Touch: Even light touch can cause pain (allodynia), and some people experience an exaggerated response to painful stimuli (hyperalgesia).
   - Loss of Coordination and Balance: Damage to sensory nerves can affect proprioception—the sense of where your body is in space—leading to clumsiness and falls.

2. Motor Symptoms:
   - Muscle Weakness: Neuropathy can cause muscles to weaken, particularly in the legs and arms, making tasks like walking or lifting objects difficult.
   - Muscle Cramps and Twitching: Uncontrolled muscle contractions and spasms can occur, leading to discomfort and fatigue.
   - Paralysis: In severe cases, nerve damage can lead to partial or complete paralysis of the affected muscles.

3. Autonomic Symptoms:
   - Digestive Issues: Autonomic neuropathy can affect the digestive system, causing symptoms such as nausea, vomiting, diarrhea, or constipation. It can also lead to difficulty swallowing.
   - Blood Pressure and Heart Rate Changes: Damage to autonomic nerves can cause erratic blood pressure and heart rate, leading to dizziness, fainting, and increased risk of heart complications.
   - Bladder and Sexual Dysfunction: Neuropathy can affect bladder control, leading to incontinence or difficulty urinating. It can also cause sexual dysfunction, such as erectile dysfunction in men and vaginal dryness in women.
   - Sweating Abnormalities: Autonomic neuropathy can disrupt normal sweating patterns, causing excessive sweating or the inability to sweat, which affects temperature regulation.

# Part 2

# The Role of Diet in Managing Peripheral Neuropathy

## *How Diet Can Influence Neuropathy*

The role of diet in managing and potentially alleviating the symptoms of peripheral neuropathy is both profound and deeply empowering. For many, the realization that food choices can influence their health and well-being offers a glimmer of hope amidst the pain and discomfort of neuropathy. This connection between diet and nerve health underscores the importance of nutrition in our lives and opens a pathway to reclaiming a sense of control over the condition. Peripheral neuropathy, with its persistent pain, tingling, and numbness, can be a daily challenge that wears down even the most resilient individuals. Yet, within the sphere of diet and nutrition lies a source of strength and potential relief. Proper nutrition not only supports overall health but can also directly impact nerve function and reduce the severity of neuropathy symptoms. It's a story of resilience, hope, and the incredible power of making mindful choices. One of the most significant ways diet influences neuropathy is through the management of blood sugar levels. For those with diabetic neuropathy, maintaining stable blood glucose levels is crucial. Consistently high blood sugar levels can damage nerves over time, leading to the painful symptoms of neuropathy. By choosing a diet rich in whole foods—such as vegetables, fruits, whole grains, and lean proteins—individuals can help keep their blood sugar levels in check. This proactive approach not only prevents further nerve damage but can also alleviate existing symptoms, offering a beacon of hope in the journey of managing diabetes and neuropathy.

Moreover, certain nutrients play pivotal roles in nerve health. For instance, B vitamins, particularly B1 (thiamine), B6 (pyridoxine), and B12 (cobalamin), are essential for nerve function and repair. Thiamine helps to convert carbohydrates into energy and is vital for nerve cell function, while pyridoxine supports neurotransmitter production, and cobalamin is crucial for the formation of the myelin sheath that protects nerve fibers. Including foods rich in these vitamins, such as whole grains, legumes, nuts, eggs, dairy products, and fortified cereals, can help nourish the nerves and support their optimal function. Antioxidants, too, have a critical role to play. Oxidative stress, which involves damage caused by free radicals, is a contributing factor to nerve damage in neuropathy. Antioxidants help neutralize these free radicals, reducing oxidative stress and potentially alleviating neuropathy symptoms. A diet abundant in colorful fruits and vegetables, such as berries, leafy greens, and bell peppers, provides a wealth of antioxidants like vitamins C and E, which are powerful allies in the fight against nerve damage.

Omega-3 fatty acids, found in fatty fish like salmon, mackerel, and sardines, as well as in flaxseeds and walnuts, are known for their anti-inflammatory properties. Chronic inflammation can exacerbate neuropathy symptoms, leading to increased pain and discomfort. By incorporating omega-3-rich foods into the diet, individuals can help reduce inflammation, potentially easing the symptoms of neuropathy and improving overall nerve health. These foods offer not just physical benefits but also a sense of proactive engagement in managing the condition. Magnesium is another nutrient that holds promise for those suffering from neuropathy. Magnesium helps regulate nerve and muscle function and may play a role in reducing neuropathic pain. Foods rich in magnesium, such as leafy green vegetables, nuts, seeds, and whole grains, can be beneficial additions to a neuropathy-friendly diet. The act of choosing these foods becomes a daily affirmation of one's commitment to health and well-being.

Dietary fiber is essential for maintaining digestive health, which can be affected by autonomic neuropathy. Foods high in fiber, such as fruits, vegetables, legumes, and whole grains, promote regular bowel movements and prevent constipation, a common issue in autonomic neuropathy. The simple act of eating a fiber-rich diet can bring comfort and regularity, providing a small but significant victory in the daily management of neuropathy. Hydration is another critical aspect of managing neuropathy through diet. Dehydration can worsen neuropathy symptoms, leading to increased pain and discomfort. Drinking plenty of water throughout the day helps keep the body and nerves hydrated, supporting overall nerve function and reducing symptoms. It's a reminder that sometimes, the simplest actions—like staying hydrated—can have a profound impact on our health.

Incorporating these dietary principles into daily life is more than just a strategy for managing neuropathy; it's a journey toward reclaiming control and finding empowerment. It's about transforming the way we view food—not merely as sustenance but as a source of healing and strength. For those living with peripheral neuropathy, every meal becomes an opportunity to nourish the body, support nerve health, and move toward a future with reduced pain and improved quality of life.

# Key Nutrients for Nerve Health

**Vitamin B1 (Thiamine)**
Thiamine, also known as vitamin B1, is essential for nerve function and energy metabolism. It helps convert carbohydrates into energy, which is vital for nerve cells' proper functioning. Thiamine also supports the health of myelin, the protective sheath that surrounds nerve fibers. Deficiency in thiamine can lead to neurological problems, including neuropathy. Good dietary sources of thiamine include whole grains, legumes, nuts, seeds, pork, and fortified cereals.

**Vitamin B6 (Pyridoxine)**
Vitamin B6 plays a critical role in nerve health by aiding in the production of neurotransmitters, which are chemicals that transmit signals in the nervous system. Pyridoxine helps maintain the health of nerve endings and supports overall nerve function. A deficiency in B6 can result in nerve damage and neuropathy. Foods rich in vitamin B6 include poultry, fish, potatoes, bananas, chickpeas, and fortified cereals.

**Vitamin B12 (Cobalamin)**
Vitamin B12 is crucial for maintaining healthy nerve cells and producing DNA and RNA. It also plays a role in forming the myelin sheath. A deficiency in vitamin B12 can lead to serious neurological issues, including peripheral neuropathy, characterized by tingling, numbness, and even muscle weakness. Dietary sources of B12 include meat, fish, dairy products, eggs, and fortified plant-based milk.

**Vitamin D**
Vitamin D, known for its role in bone health, also supports nerve health. It helps regulate the immune system and reduce inflammation, which can benefit those with neuropathic pain. Some studies suggest that low levels of vitamin D are associated with an increased risk of developing neuropathy. Sources of vitamin D include sunlight exposure, fatty fish like salmon and mackerel, fortified dairy products, and supplements.

**Vitamin E**
Vitamin E is a powerful antioxidant that helps protect nerve cells from damage caused by free radicals. It plays a significant role in maintaining the integrity of cell membranes and overall nerve health. A deficiency in vitamin E can lead to neurological problems, including peripheral neuropathy. Good sources of vitamin E include nuts, seeds, spinach, broccoli, and vegetable oils such as sunflower and safflower oil.

**Omega-3 Fatty Acids**
Omega-3 fatty acids, particularly EPA and DHA, are essential for reducing inflammation and supporting nerve function. These fatty acids help maintain the structure and function of nerve cell membranes, promoting healthy communication between nerve cells. Omega-3s are found in fatty fish such as salmon, mackerel, and sardines, as well as in flaxseeds, chia seeds, and walnuts.

### Magnesium
Magnesium plays a vital role in nerve transmission and muscle contraction. It helps regulate calcium levels in the nerve cells, ensuring proper nerve function and preventing overstimulation that can lead to neuropathic pain. Magnesium deficiency can exacerbate neuropathy symptoms. Foods rich in magnesium include leafy green vegetables, nuts, seeds, whole grains, and legumes.

### Alpha-Lipoic Acid
Alpha-lipoic acid (ALA) is a potent antioxidant that helps reduce oxidative stress and inflammation in the nerves. It also aids in the regeneration of other antioxidants, enhancing overall nerve health. ALA has been shown to improve symptoms of peripheral neuropathy, especially in diabetic patients. Sources of alpha-lipoic acid include spinach, broccoli, potatoes, and organ meats, though it is often taken as a supplement for therapeutic purposes.

### Acetyl-L-Carnitine
Acetyl-L-carnitine is an amino acid that helps produce energy in cells and has neuroprotective properties. It supports the regeneration of damaged nerves and has been shown to reduce pain and improve nerve function in individuals with neuropathy. Dietary sources of acetyl-L-carnitine include meat, fish, poultry, and dairy products, though it is also commonly taken as a supplement.

### Zinc
Zinc is essential for maintaining a healthy immune system and supporting nerve function. It plays a role in cell growth, DNA synthesis, and the repair of nerve tissues. Zinc deficiency can impair nerve health and contribute to neuropathy symptoms. Good sources of zinc include meat, shellfish, legumes, seeds, nuts, and dairy products.

### Curcumin
Curcumin, the active compound in turmeric, has powerful anti-inflammatory and antioxidant properties. It helps protect nerves from damage and reduce inflammation that can contribute to neuropathic pain. Incorporating turmeric into the diet or taking curcumin supplements can be beneficial for nerve health. Turmeric can be used in cooking or taken as a supplement.

### Integrating These Nutrients into Your Diet
Understanding the importance of these key nutrients is the first step; the next is integrating them into your daily diet. Here are some practical tips:
- Balanced Meals: Aim for balanced meals that include a variety of food groups. Incorporate whole grains, lean proteins, healthy fats, and plenty of fruits and vegetables.
- Diverse Sources: Get these nutrients from diverse sources to ensure a wide range of vitamins and minerals. For example, include different types of fish, nuts, seeds, and vegetables in your meals.

- Supplements: If necessary, consider supplements to fill nutritional gaps, especially if you have dietary restrictions or deficiencies. Always consult with a healthcare provider before starting any supplements.
- Healthy Cooking Methods: Use healthy cooking methods such as grilling, baking, steaming, and sautéing with minimal oil to preserve nutrient content and enhance flavors.

# Foods to Avoid

When managing peripheral neuropathy, diet plays a crucial role not only in alleviating symptoms but also in preventing further nerve damage. While certain nutrients and foods can support nerve health, there are also foods that can exacerbate neuropathy symptoms and contribute to overall nerve degeneration. Knowing which foods to avoid is just as important as knowing which foods to include in your diet. Here is a comprehensive look at the foods that should be minimized or eliminated to help manage peripheral neuropathy effectively.

**Sugary Foods and Beverages**
High sugar intake is detrimental to nerve health, particularly for individuals with diabetic neuropathy. Consuming excessive sugar can lead to spikes in blood glucose levels, causing inflammation and oxidative stress, both of which can damage nerves. Furthermore, high blood sugar levels over time can exacerbate diabetic neuropathy, increasing pain and discomfort.

- Avoid: Sweets, candies, sugary cereals, desserts, sodas, fruit juices with added sugar, and other sugar-laden beverages.
- Opt for: Natural sweeteners like stevia or monk fruit, and satisfy your sweet tooth with fresh fruits, which offer fiber and nutrients alongside natural sugars.

**Refined Carbohydrates**
Refined carbohydrates, such as white bread, white rice, and pasta, can have a similar effect on blood sugar levels as sugary foods. They are quickly broken down into glucose, causing rapid spikes in blood sugar and insulin levels. This can lead to increased inflammation and nerve damage over time.

- Avoid: White bread, white rice, regular pasta, pastries, and other processed grains.
- Opt for: Whole grains like brown rice, quinoa, whole wheat bread, and whole grain pasta, which have a lower glycemic index and provide more fiber and nutrients.

**Trans Fats and Saturated Fats**
Trans fats and saturated fats contribute to inflammation and cardiovascular problems, which can indirectly affect nerve health. Trans fats, often found in processed and fried foods, are particularly harmful and have been linked to increased inflammation and insulin resistance. Saturated fats, primarily found in animal products, can also exacerbate inflammation if consumed in large amounts.

- Avoid: Fried foods, margarine, shortening, commercially baked goods (like cookies, crackers, and cakes), fatty cuts of meat, and full-fat dairy products.
- Opt for: Healthy fats such as those found in olive oil, avocados, nuts, seeds, and fatty fish like salmon and mackerel.

**Processed and Packaged Foods**

Processed and packaged foods often contain high levels of sodium, unhealthy fats, preservatives, and artificial additives, all of which can contribute to inflammation and poor overall health. These foods are typically low in essential nutrients needed for nerve repair and maintenance.

- Avoid: Packaged snacks, ready-to-eat meals, processed meats (like sausages and deli meats), and canned soups with high sodium content.
- Opt for: Fresh, whole foods, and prepare meals at home where you can control the ingredients and cooking methods.

**Alcohol**

Chronic alcohol consumption can lead to nutritional deficiencies, particularly of B vitamins, which are crucial for nerve health. Alcohol itself is neurotoxic, and excessive intake can directly damage nerve tissues, exacerbating neuropathy symptoms and increasing the risk of developing alcoholic neuropathy.

- Avoid: Alcoholic beverages, including beer, wine, and spirits.
- Opt for: Non-alcoholic beverages such as water, herbal teas, and naturally flavored seltzers. If you choose to drink alcohol, do so in moderation and consult your healthcare provider.

**Foods High in Sodium**

High sodium intake can lead to high blood pressure, which can damage blood vessels, including those that supply blood to the nerves. Poor blood circulation can exacerbate neuropathy symptoms and lead to further nerve damage.

- Avoid: Salty snacks, canned and processed foods, pickles, and fast food.
- Opt for: Fresh, whole foods with minimal added salt. Use herbs and spices to flavor your food instead of relying on salt.

**Artificial Sweeteners**

While artificial sweeteners are often used as a sugar substitute, some studies suggest they may have negative effects on nerve health and overall metabolism. Certain artificial sweeteners have been linked to increased inflammation and adverse effects on glucose metabolism.

- Avoid: Artificial sweeteners like aspartame, saccharin, and sucralose.
- Opt for: Natural sweeteners like stevia, monk fruit, and small amounts of honey or maple syrup, used in moderation.

**Caffeine**

While moderate caffeine consumption can be part of a healthy diet, excessive caffeine intake can interfere with sleep patterns, which is crucial for nerve repair and overall health. Poor sleep can exacerbate neuropathy symptoms and reduce the body's ability to heal.

- Avoid: Excessive consumption of coffee, energy drinks, and caffeinated sodas.
- Opt for: Limiting caffeine intake to moderate levels, and considering herbal teas or decaffeinated beverages as alternatives.

# Breakfast Recipes

**1. Avocado Toast with Poached Egg**
**Servings: 2**
**Cooking Time: 15 minutes**
**Ingredients**

- 2 slices of whole grain bread
- 1 ripe avocado
- 2 large eggs
- 1 tablespoon lemon juice
- 1 teaspoon olive oil
- 1/4 teaspoon paprika
- 1/4 teaspoon garlic powder
- Freshly ground black pepper
- Fresh herbs (optional, for garnish, such as parsley or cilantro)

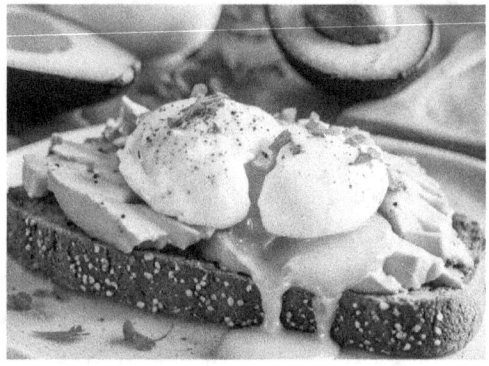

**Instructions**

1. Prepare the Avocado Spread:
   - Halve the avocado, remove the pit, and scoop the flesh into a bowl.
   - Add the lemon juice, olive oil, paprika, garlic powder, and black pepper. Mash until smooth and well combined.
2. Toast the Bread:
   - Toast the slices of whole grain bread to your desired level of crispiness.
3. Poach the Eggs:
   - Bring a medium pot of water to a gentle simmer.
   - Crack each egg into a small bowl.
   - Create a gentle whirlpool in the pot using a spoon and carefully slide the eggs into the water one at a time.
   - Poach the eggs for about 3-4 minutes, or until the whites are set and the yolks are still runny.
   - Use a slotted spoon to remove the eggs from the water and set them on a plate.
4. Assemble the Toast:
   - Spread the mashed avocado mixture evenly over the toasted bread slices.
   - Top each slice with a poached egg.
   - Garnish with freshly ground black pepper and fresh herbs, if desired.

**Nutrition Info (per serving)**

- Calories: 300   Protein: 12g   Carbohydrates: 22g   Fiber: 8g
- Sugars: 2g   Total Fat: 20g   Saturated Fat: 3g
- Cholesterol: 190mg
- Sodium: 120mg

## 2. Quinoa Porridge

**Servings:** 2
**Cooking Time:** 25 minutes

**Ingredients**
- 1/2 cup quinoa
- 1 cup unsweetened almond milk (or any preferred non-dairy milk)
- 1/2 cup water
- 1 tablespoon chia seeds
- 1 teaspoon ground cinnamon
- 1 teaspoon vanilla extract
- 2 tablespoons maple syrup
- Fresh fruit (such as berries, banana slices, or apple slices) for topping

**Instructions**
1. Rinse the Quinoa:
   - Rinse the quinoa under cold water using a fine-mesh sieve to remove any bitterness.
2. Cook the Quinoa:
   - In a medium saucepan, combine the rinsed quinoa, almond milk, and water. Bring to a boil over medium-high heat.
   - Reduce the heat to low, cover, and simmer for about 15 minutes, or until the quinoa is tender and has absorbed most of the liquid.
3. Add Flavorings:
   - Stir in the chia seeds, ground cinnamon, vanilla extract, and maple syrup.
   - Continue to cook for another 5 minutes, stirring occasionally, until the porridge thickens to your desired consistency.
4. Serve:
   - Divide the quinoa porridge into two bowls.
   - Top with fresh fruit of your choice.

**Nutrition Info (per serving)**
- Calories: 260
- Protein: 8g
- Carbohydrates: 45g
- Fiber: 7g
- Sugars: 14g
- Total Fat: 6g
- Saturated Fat: 0.5g
- Cholesterol: 0mg
- Sodium: 60mg

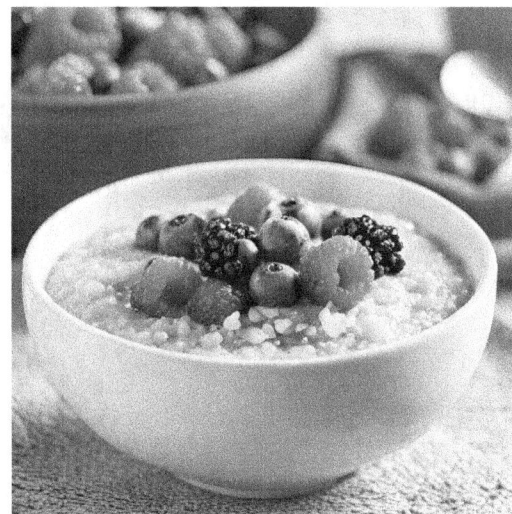

## 3. Oatmeal with Mixed Berries

**Servings:** 2
**Cooking Time:** 10 minutes

**Ingredients**
- 1 cup rolled oats
- 2 cups water or unsweetened almond milk (or any preferred non-dairy milk)
- 1 teaspoon ground cinnamon
- 1 teaspoon vanilla extract
- 1 tablespoon flaxseeds
- 1 cup mixed berries (fresh or frozen)
- 2 tablespoons chopped nuts (such as almonds or walnuts)
- 1 tablespoon honey (optional)

**Instructions**
1. Cook the Oats:
   - In a medium saucepan, bring the water or almond milk to a boil.
   - Add the rolled oats, reduce the heat to low, and simmer for about 5 minutes, stirring occasionally, until the oats are tender and the mixture has thickened.
2. Add Flavorings:
   - Stir in the ground cinnamon, vanilla extract, and flaxseeds.
3. Serve:
   - Divide the oatmeal into two bowls.
   - Top with mixed berries and chopped nuts.
   - Drizzle with honey, if desired.

**Nutrition Info (per serving)**
- Calories: 320
- Protein: 9g
- Carbohydrates: 53g
- Fiber: 9g
- Sugars: 13g
- Total Fat: 10g
- Saturated Fat: 1g
- Cholesterol: 0mg
- Sodium: 10mg

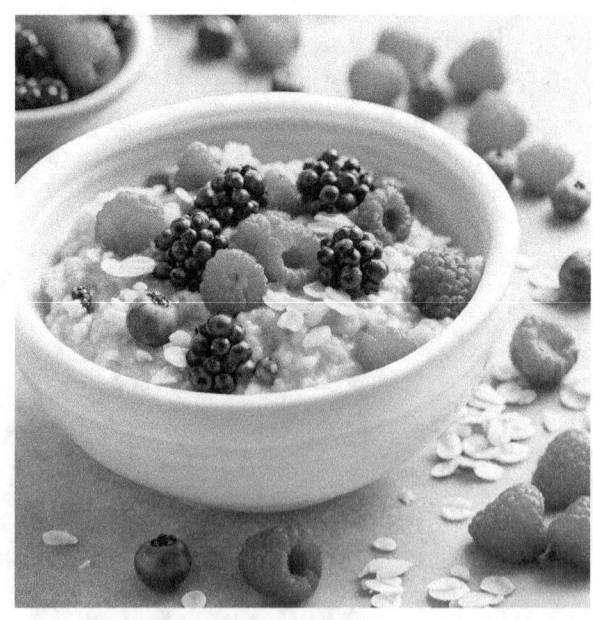

## 4. Smoothie Bowl

**Servings:** 2
**Cooking Time: 10 minutes**

**Ingredients**

- 1 banana, frozen
- 1 cup frozen berries (such as blueberries, strawberries, or raspberries)
- 1/2 cup unsweetened almond milk (or any preferred non-dairy milk)
- 1 tablespoon chia seeds
- 1 teaspoon vanilla extract
- **Toppings:**
    - Fresh fruit slices (such as kiwi, banana, or mango)
    - Granola
    - Coconut flakes
    - Chopped nuts (such as almonds or pecans)

**Instructions**

1. Blend the Smoothie:
    - In a blender, combine the frozen banana, frozen berries, almond milk, chia seeds, and vanilla extract.
    - Blend until smooth and creamy, adding more almond milk if necessary to achieve the desired consistency.
2. Serve:
    - Pour the smoothie into two bowls.
    - Top with fresh fruit slices, granola, coconut flakes, and chopped nuts.

**Nutrition Info (per serving)**

- Calories: 280
- Protein: 5g
- Carbohydrates: 50g
- Fiber: 10g
- Sugars: 25g
- Total Fat: 8g
- Saturated Fat: 2g
- Cholesterol: 0mg
- Sodium: 60mg

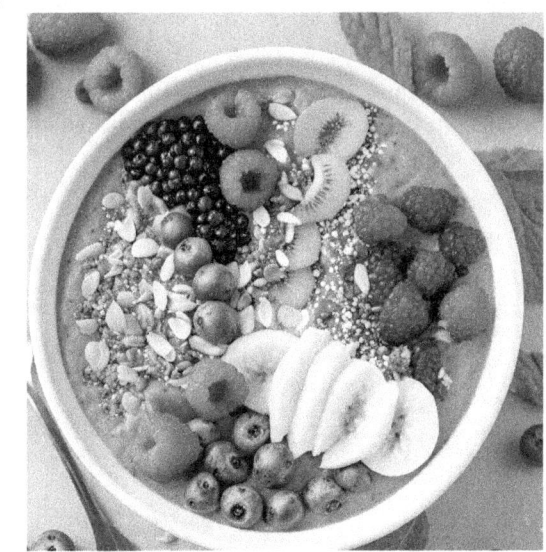

## 5. Vegetable Omelet

**Servings:** 2
**Cooking Time:** 15 minutes

### Ingredients
- 4 large eggs
- 1/4 cup unsweetened almond milk (or any preferred non-dairy milk)
- 1/2 cup diced bell peppers (any color)
- 1/2 cup diced tomatoes
- 1/2 cup chopped spinach
- 1/4 cup chopped onions
- 1 tablespoon olive oil
- 1/4 teaspoon turmeric
- Freshly ground black pepper
- Fresh herbs (optional, for garnish, such as parsley or chives)

### Instructions
1. Prepare the Egg Mixture:
   - In a bowl, whisk together the eggs, almond milk, turmeric, and black pepper until well combined.
2. Cook the Vegetables:
   - In a non-stick skillet, heat the olive oil over medium heat.
   - Add the onions, bell peppers, and tomatoes. Sauté for 3-4 minutes until the vegetables are tender.
   - Add the spinach and cook for another 1-2 minutes until wilted.
3. Cook the Omelet:
   - Pour the egg mixture over the cooked vegetables in the skillet.
   - Cook for 4-5 minutes, or until the eggs are set and the omelet is firm.
   - Carefully fold the omelet in half and cook for another minute.
4. Serve:
   - Cut the omelet in half and serve each half on a plate.
   - Garnish with fresh herbs if desired.

### Nutrition Info (per serving)
- Calories: 230
- Protein: 15g
- Carbohydrates: 6g
- Fiber: 2g
- Sugars: 3g
- Total Fat: 16g
- Saturated Fat: 4g
- Cholesterol: 375mg
- Sodium: 130mg

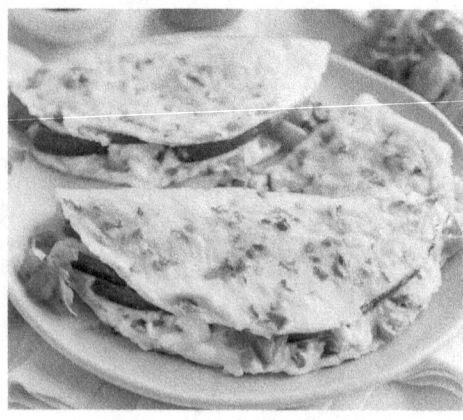

## 6. Banana Pancakes
**Servings:** 2
**Cooking Time:** 20 minutes
**Ingredients**
- 2 ripe bananas
- 2 large eggs
- 1/2 cup rolled oats
- 1/2 teaspoon baking powder
- 1 teaspoon vanilla extract
- 1 teaspoon ground cinnamon
- 1 tablespoon coconut oil (for cooking)
- Fresh fruit and chopped nuts for topping

**Instructions**
1. Prepare the Batter:
   - In a blender, combine the bananas, eggs, rolled oats, baking powder, vanilla extract, and ground cinnamon. Blend until smooth.
2. Cook the Pancakes:
   - Heat a non-stick skillet over medium heat and add a small amount of coconut oil.
   - Pour small amounts of batter onto the skillet to form pancakes (about 1/4 cup each).
   - Cook for 2-3 minutes on each side, or until bubbles form on the surface and the edges are set.
3. Serve:
   - Stack the pancakes on plates.
   - Top with fresh fruit and chopped nuts.

**Nutrition Info (per serving)**
- Calories: 290
- Protein: 10g
- Carbohydrates: 45g
- Fiber: 5g
- Sugars: 14g
- Total Fat: 10g
- Saturated Fat: 3g
- Cholesterol: 185mg
- Sodium: 110mg

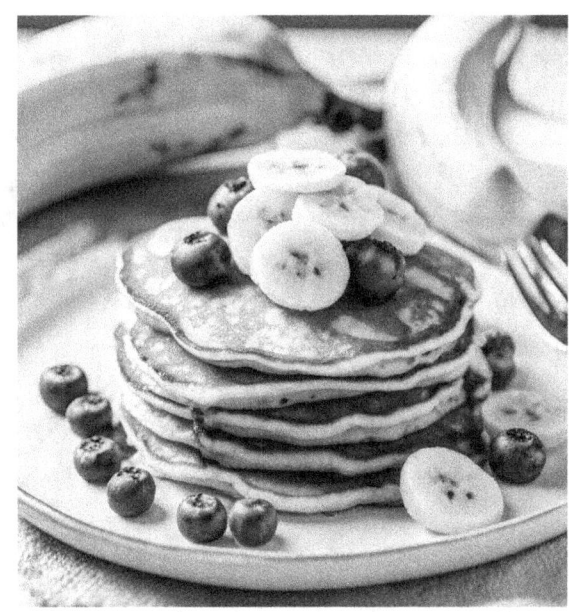

## 7. Sweet Potato Hash

**Servings:** 2
**Cooking Time:** 25 minutes

**Ingredients**
- 2 medium sweet potatoes, peeled and diced
- 1 red bell pepper, diced
- 1 green bell pepper, diced
- 1 small onion, chopped
- 2 tablespoons olive oil
- 1/2 teaspoon smoked paprika
- 1/4 teaspoon ground cumin
- Freshly ground black pepper
- Fresh parsley (optional, for garnish)

**Instructions**

1. Cook the Sweet Potatoes:
   - In a large skillet, heat 1 tablespoon of olive oil over medium heat.
   - Add the diced sweet potatoes and cook for about 10 minutes, stirring occasionally, until they begin to soften.
2. Add Vegetables and Spices:
   - Add the remaining olive oil, bell peppers, and onion to the skillet.
   - Cook for another 10-15 minutes, stirring occasionally, until the vegetables are tender and the sweet potatoes are golden brown.
   - Stir in the smoked paprika, ground cumin, and black pepper.
3. Serve:
   - Divide the sweet potato hash onto plates.
   - Garnish with fresh parsley if desired.

**Nutrition Info (per serving)**
- Calories: 240
- Protein: 3g
- Carbohydrates: 38g
- Fiber: 7g
- Sugars: 9g
- Total Fat: 10g
- Saturated Fat: 1.5g
- Cholesterol: 0mg
- Sodium: 65mg

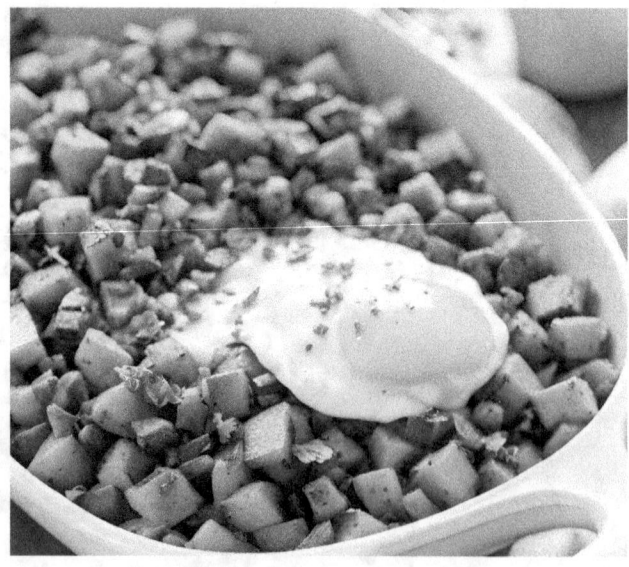

# 8. Nutty Rice Pudding

**Servings:** 2
**Cooking Time:** 40 minutes

**Ingredients**

- 1/2 cup brown rice
- 2 cups unsweetened almond milk (or any preferred non-dairy milk)
- 1/4 cup raisins
- 1 teaspoon ground cinnamon
- 1 teaspoon vanilla extract
- 2 tablespoons chopped nuts (such as almonds or walnuts)
- 1 tablespoon honey (optional)

**Instructions**

1. Cook the Rice:
   - In a medium saucepan, combine the brown rice and almond milk.
   - Bring to a boil over medium-high heat, then reduce the heat to low, cover, and simmer for about 30 minutes, or until the rice is tender and most of the liquid is absorbed.
2. Add Flavorings and Raisins:
   - Stir in the raisins, ground cinnamon, and vanilla extract.
   - Cook for another 5-10 minutes, stirring occasionally, until the mixture thickens to your desired consistency.
3. Serve:
   - Divide the rice pudding into bowls.
   - Top with chopped nuts and drizzle with honey if desired.

**Nutrition Info (per serving)**

- Calories: 280
- Protein: 6g
- Carbohydrates: 49g
- Fiber: 4g
- Sugars: 19g
- Total Fat: 8g
- Saturated Fat: 0.5g
- Cholesterol: 0mg
- Sodium: 80mg

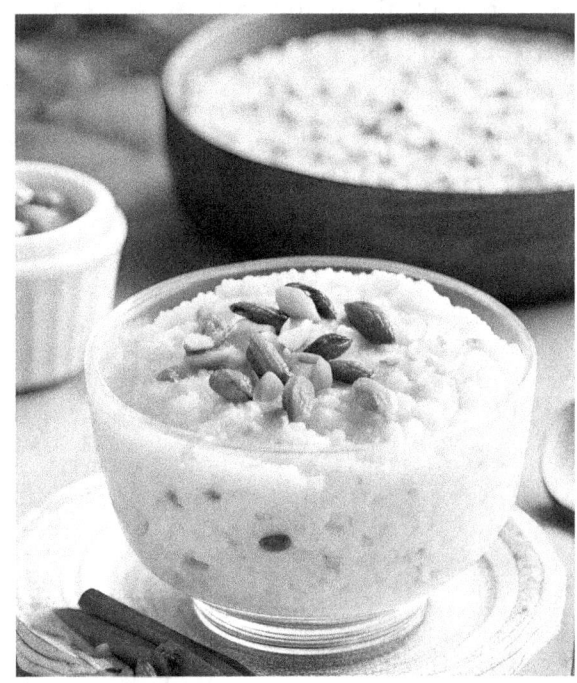

## 9. Buckwheat Crepes

**Servings:** 4
**Cooking Time:** 30 minutes

**Ingredients**
- 1 cup buckwheat flour
- 2 large eggs
- 1 1/4 cups unsweetened almond milk (or any preferred non-dairy milk)
- 1 tablespoon melted coconut oil
- 1 teaspoon vanilla extract
- Fresh fruit, yogurt, and nuts for topping

**Instructions**
1. Prepare the Batter:
   - In a bowl, whisk together the buckwheat flour, eggs, almond milk, melted coconut oil, and vanilla extract until smooth.
   - Let the batter rest for 10 minutes.
2. Cook the Crepes:
   - Heat a non-stick skillet over medium heat and lightly grease with coconut oil.
   - Pour a small amount of batter into the skillet and swirl to spread evenly.
   - Cook for 1-2 minutes on each side, or until the edges are golden brown and the crepe is set.
   - Repeat with the remaining batter.
3. Serve:
   - Stack the crepes on plates.
   - Top with fresh fruit, yogurt, and nuts.

**Nutrition Info (per serving)**
- Calories: 150
- Protein: 6g
- Carbohydrates: 22g
- Fiber: 3g
- Sugars: 3g
- Total Fat: 5g
- Saturated Fat: 2g
- Cholesterol: 55mg
- Sodium: 45mg

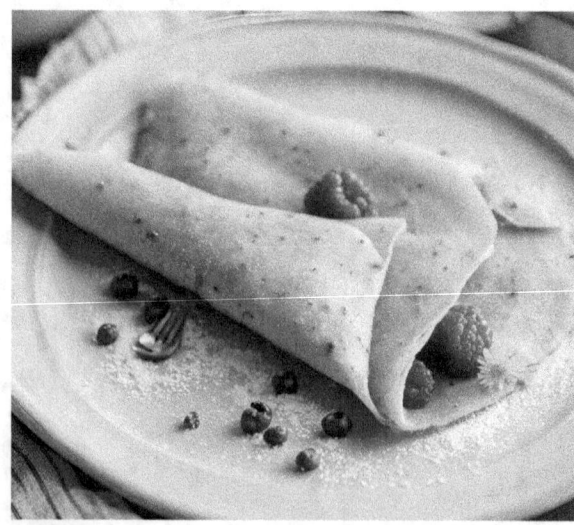

## 10. Muesli and Yogurt

**Servings:** 2
**Cooking Time:** 5 minutes

**Ingredients**
- 1 cup rolled oats
- 1/4 cup chopped nuts (such as almonds, walnuts, or hazelnuts)
- 1/4 cup dried fruit (such as raisins, apricots, or cranberries)
- 1 tablespoon chia seeds
- 1 teaspoon ground cinnamon
- 1 cup plain Greek yogurt (or any preferred non-dairy yogurt)
- Fresh fruit for topping (such as berries or sliced banana)
- 1 tablespoon honey (optional)

**Instructions**
1. Prepare the Muesli:
    - In a large bowl, combine the rolled oats, chopped nuts, dried fruit, chia seeds, and ground cinnamon. Mix well.
2. Serve:
    - Divide the Greek yogurt into two bowls.
    - Top each bowl with the muesli mixture and fresh fruit.
    - Drizzle with honey if desired.

**Nutrition Info (per serving)**
- Calories: 350
- Protein: 14g
- Carbohydrates: 55g
- Fiber: 8g
- Sugars: 20g
- Total Fat: 10g
- Saturated Fat: 2g
- Cholesterol: 0mg
- Sodium: 70mg

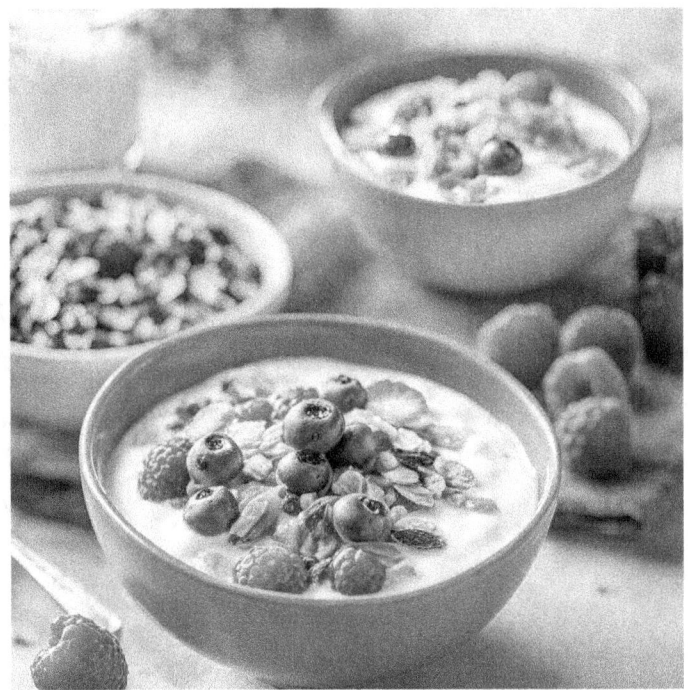

## 11. Spinach and Feta Wrap

**Servings:** 2
**Cooking Time:** 10 minutes

**Ingredients**
- 2 whole grain tortillas
- 1 cup fresh spinach leaves
- 1/2 cup crumbled feta cheese
- 1/4 cup chopped sun-dried tomatoes (not in oil)
- 1 tablespoon olive oil
- 1 teaspoon dried oregano
- Freshly ground black pepper

**Instructions**
1. Prepare the Filling:
   - In a skillet, heat the olive oil over medium heat.
   - Add the spinach and sauté for 2-3 minutes until wilted.
   - Stir in the sun-dried tomatoes, feta cheese, oregano, and black pepper. Cook for another 1-2 minutes until heated through.
2. Assemble the Wraps:
   - Lay out the tortillas and divide the spinach mixture evenly between them.
   - Roll up the tortillas, folding in the sides as you go.
3. Serve:
   - Cut each wrap in half and serve warm.

**Nutrition Info (per serving)**
- Calories: 290
- Protein: 10g
- Carbohydrates: 28g
- Fiber: 4g
- Sugars: 2g
- Total Fat: 16g
- Saturated Fat: 5g
- Cholesterol: 25mg
- Sodium: 470mg

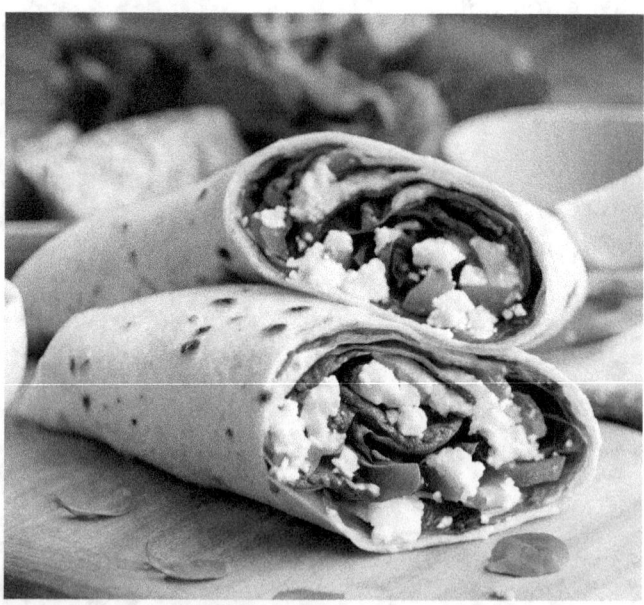

## 12. Almond Butter and Banana Sandwich

**Servings:** 2
**Cooking Time:** 5 minutes

**Ingredients**
- 4 slices of whole grain bread
- 4 tablespoons almond butter
- 2 bananas, sliced
- 1 tablespoon chia seeds
- 1 teaspoon ground cinnamon

**Instructions**
1. Prepare the Sandwiches:
    - Spread 2 tablespoons of almond butter on two slices of bread.
    - Arrange the banana slices evenly over the almond butter.
    - Sprinkle chia seeds and ground cinnamon on top of the bananas.
    - Top with the remaining slices of bread.
2. Serve:
    - Cut each sandwich in half and serve immediately.

**Nutrition Info (per serving)**
- Calories: 360
- Protein: 10g
- Carbohydrates: 52g
- Fiber: 8g
- Sugars: 15g
- Total Fat: 14g
- Saturated Fat: 1g
- Cholesterol: 0mg
- Sodium: 140mg

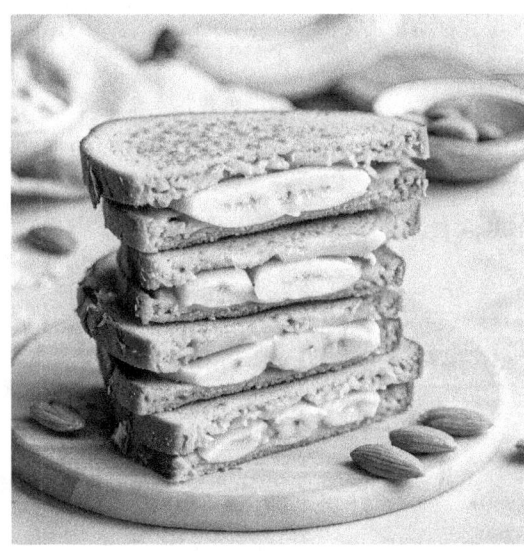

## 13. Egg Muffins

**Servings:** 6 (2 muffins per serving)
**Cooking Time:** 25 minutes

### Ingredients
- 10 large eggs
- 1 cup chopped spinach
- 1/2 cup diced bell peppers (any color)
- 1/4 cup diced onions
- 1/4 cup crumbled feta cheese
- 1 teaspoon dried basil
- Freshly ground black pepper
- 1 tablespoon olive oil (for greasing the muffin tin)

### Instructions
1. Preheat Oven:
   - Preheat your oven to 375°F (190°C).
   - Grease a 12-cup muffin tin with olive oil.
2. Prepare the Egg Mixture:
   - In a large bowl, whisk the eggs until well combined.
   - Stir in the spinach, bell peppers, onions, feta cheese, dried basil, and black pepper.
3. Fill the Muffin Tin:
   - Pour the egg mixture evenly into the prepared muffin cups, filling each about three-quarters full.
4. Bake:
   - Bake for 20 minutes, or until the egg muffins are set and lightly golden on top.
5. Serve:
   - Let the muffins cool for a few minutes before removing them from the tin.
   - Serve warm.

### Nutrition Info (per serving)
- Calories: 150
- Protein: 12g
- Carbohydrates: 3g
- Fiber: 1g
- Sugars: 1g
- Total Fat: 10g
- Saturated Fat: 3g
- Cholesterol: 275mg
- Sodium: 200mg

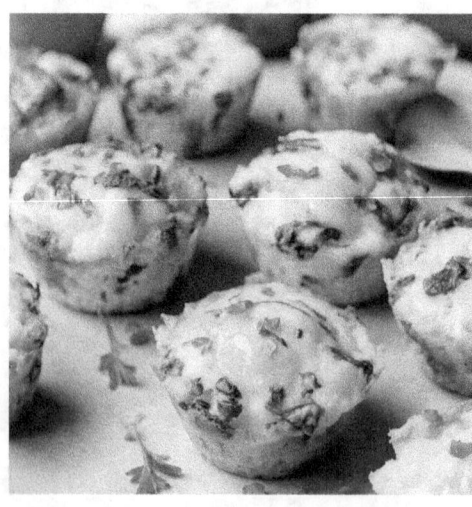

## 14. Tofu Scramble

**Servings:** 2
**Cooking Time:** 15 minutes

**Ingredients**

- 1 block (14 ounces) firm tofu, drained and crumbled
- 1 tablespoon olive oil
- 1/2 cup diced bell peppers (any color)
- 1/4 cup diced onions
- 1 cup chopped spinach
- 1 teaspoon ground turmeric
- 1/2 teaspoon garlic powder
- Freshly ground black pepper
- Fresh herbs (optional, for garnish)

**Instructions**

1. Prepare the Vegetables:
   - In a skillet, heat the olive oil over medium heat.
   - Add the diced bell peppers and onions. Sauté for 3-4 minutes until they begin to soften.
2. Cook the Tofu:
   - Add the crumbled tofu to the skillet. Cook for 5-7 minutes, stirring occasionally, until the tofu is heated through and slightly browned.
3. Add Seasonings and Spinach:
   - Stir in the ground turmeric, garlic powder, and black pepper.
   - Add the chopped spinach and cook for another 2-3 minutes until wilted.
4. Serve:
   - Divide the tofu scramble onto plates.
   - Garnish with fresh herbs if desired.

**Nutrition Info (per serving)**

- Calories: 240
- Protein: 20g
- Carbohydrates: 8g
- Fiber: 3g
- Sugars: 3g
- Total Fat: 14g
- Saturated Fat: 2g
- Cholesterol: 0mg
- Sodium: 190mg

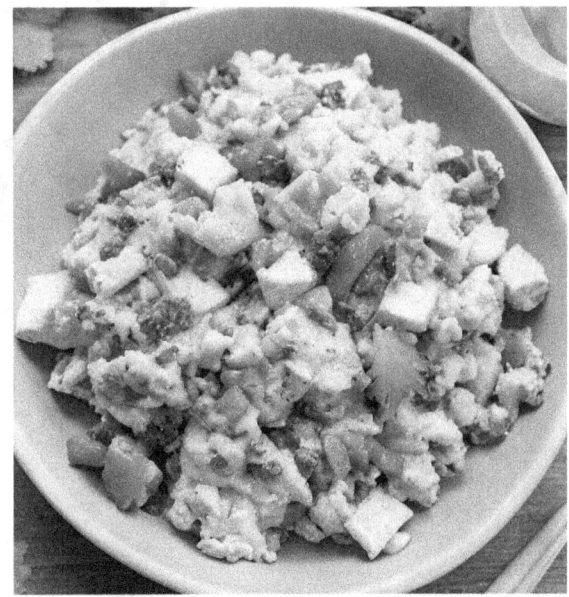

## 15. Pumpkin Oatmeal

**Servings:** 2
**Cooking Time:** 10 minutes

**Ingredients**
- 1 cup rolled oats
- 2 cups unsweetened almond milk (or any preferred non-dairy milk)
- 1/2 cup canned pumpkin puree
- 1 teaspoon ground cinnamon
- 1/2 teaspoon ground nutmeg
- 1 tablespoon chia seeds
- 2 tablespoons maple syrup
- 2 tablespoons chopped nuts (such as pecans or walnuts)

**Instructions**
1. Cook the Oats:
   - In a medium saucepan, bring the almond milk to a boil.
   - Add the rolled oats, reduce the heat to low, and simmer for about 5 minutes, stirring occasionally, until the oats are tender and the mixture has thickened.
2. Add Pumpkin and Spices:
   - Stir in the pumpkin puree, ground cinnamon, ground nutmeg, and chia seeds.
   - Cook for another 2-3 minutes, stirring frequently, until well combined and heated through.
3. Serve:
   - Divide the pumpkin oatmeal into two bowls.
   - Drizzle with maple syrup and sprinkle with chopped nuts.

**Nutrition Info (per serving)**
- Calories: 320
- Protein: 7g
- Carbohydrates: 52g
- Fiber: 8g
- Sugars: 15g
- Total Fat: 10g
- Saturated Fat: 1g
- Cholesterol: 0mg
- Sodium: 50mg

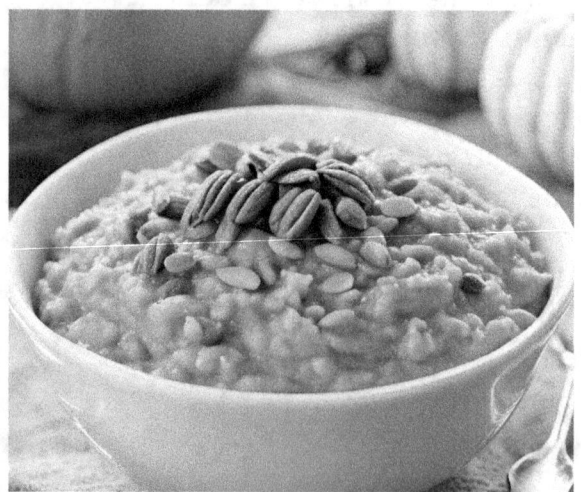

# 16. Turkey Sausage and Veggie Skillet

**Servings:** 2
**Cooking Time:** 20 minutes

## Ingredients

- 4 ounces turkey sausage, sliced
- 1 red bell pepper, diced
- 1 yellow bell pepper, diced
- 1 small zucchini, diced
- 1 small onion, chopped
- 1 tablespoon olive oil
- 1 teaspoon dried oregano
- 1/2 teaspoon garlic powder
- Freshly ground black pepper
- Fresh parsley (optional, for garnish)

## Instructions

1. Cook the Sausage:
   - In a large skillet, heat the olive oil over medium heat.
   - Add the turkey sausage slices and cook for 5-7 minutes until browned.
2. Add Vegetables and Seasonings:
   - Add the bell peppers, zucchini, and onion to the skillet.
   - Cook for another 8-10 minutes until the vegetables are tender.
   - Stir in the oregano, garlic powder, and black pepper.
3. Serve:
   - Divide the skillet mixture onto plates.
   - Garnish with fresh parsley if desired.

## Nutrition Info (per serving)

- Calories: 220
- Protein: 16g
- Carbohydrates: 12g
- Fiber: 3g
- Sugars: 6g
- Total Fat: 12g
- Saturated Fat: 3g
- Cholesterol: 55mg
- Sodium: 480mg

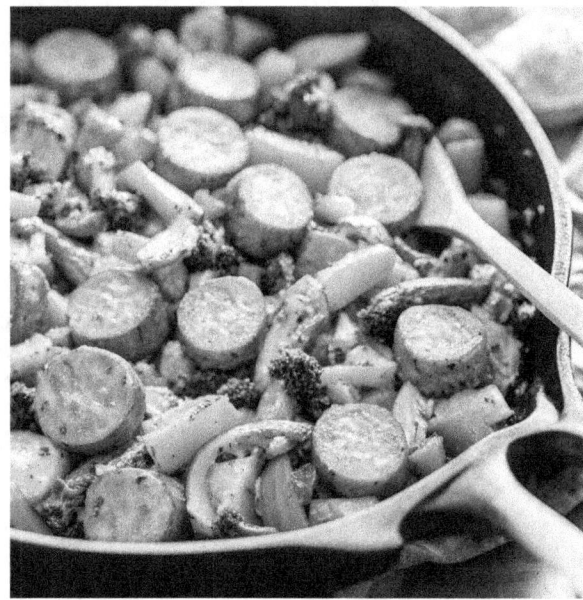

## 17. Ricotta and Tomato Toast

**Servings:** 2
**Cooking Time:** 10 minutes

**Ingredients**
- 2 slices of whole grain bread
- 1/2 cup ricotta cheese
- 1 cup cherry tomatoes, halved
- 1 tablespoon olive oil
- 1 teaspoon dried basil
- Freshly ground black pepper

**Instructions**
1. Toast the Bread:
   - Toast the slices of whole grain bread to your desired level of crispiness.
2. Prepare the Topping:
   - In a small bowl, combine the cherry tomatoes, olive oil, dried basil, and black pepper. Mix well.
3. Assemble the Toast:
   - Spread the ricotta cheese evenly over the toasted bread slices.
   - Top with the tomato mixture.
4. Serve:
   - Serve the toast immediately.

**Nutrition Info (per serving)**
- Calories: 260
- Protein: 12g
- Carbohydrates: 24g
- Fiber: 4g
- Sugars: 6g
- Total Fat: 12g
- Saturated Fat: 4g
- Cholesterol: 20mg
- Sodium: 240mg

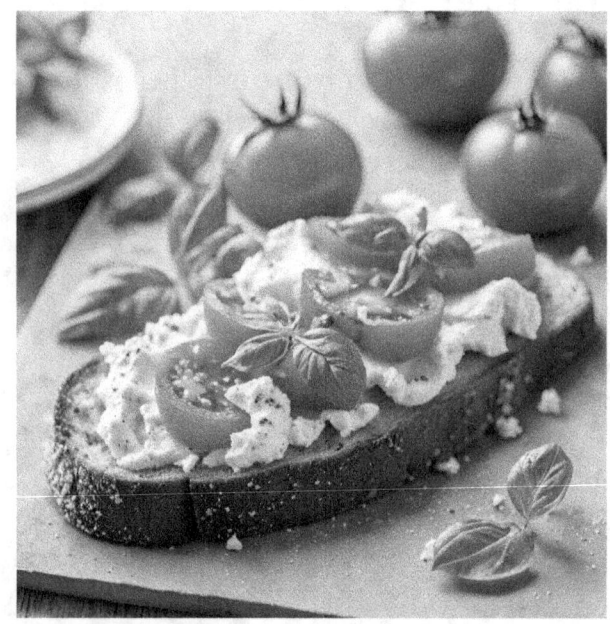

## 18. Breakfast Lentils

**Servings:** 2
**Cooking Time:** 30 minutes

### Ingredients

- 1 cup cooked green or brown lentils
- 1/2 cup diced tomatoes
- 1/4 cup diced bell peppers
- 1/4 cup chopped spinach
- 1 small onion, chopped
- 1 tablespoon olive oil
- 1 teaspoon ground cumin
- 1/2 teaspoon turmeric
- Freshly ground black pepper
- Fresh cilantro (optional, for garnish)

### Instructions

1. Prepare the Vegetables:
   - In a skillet, heat the olive oil over medium heat.
   - Add the onion and cook for 3-4 minutes until softened.
   - Add the bell peppers, tomatoes, and spinach. Cook for another 5 minutes until the vegetables are tender.
2. Add Lentils and Spices:
   - Stir in the cooked lentils, ground cumin, turmeric, and black pepper.
   - Cook for another 5-7 minutes until heated through and well combined.
3. Serve:
   - Divide the lentil mixture onto plates.
   - Garnish with fresh cilantro if desired.

### Nutrition Info (per serving)

- Calories: 240
- Protein: 12g
- Carbohydrates: 30g
- Fiber: 12g
- Sugars: 4g
- Total Fat: 8g
- Saturated Fat: 1g
- Cholesterol: 0mg
- Sodium: 120mg

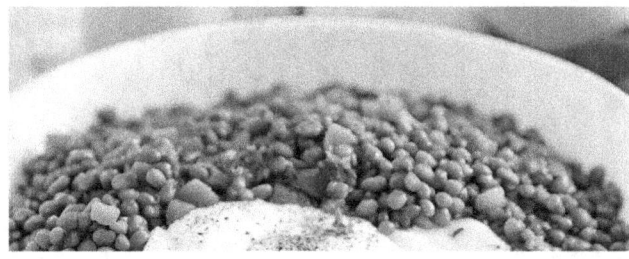

## 19. Mango and Coconut Rice

**Servings:** 2
**Cooking Time:** 20 minutes

**Ingredients**
- 1 cup cooked jasmine rice
- 1/2 cup coconut milk
- 1 tablespoon maple syrup
- 1 teaspoon vanilla extract
- 1 ripe mango, diced
- 2 tablespoons unsweetened shredded coconut
- Fresh mint leaves (optional, for garnish)

**Instructions**

1. Prepare the Rice:
   - In a medium saucepan, combine the cooked jasmine rice, coconut milk, maple syrup, and vanilla extract.
   - Cook over medium heat for 5-7 minutes, stirring frequently, until the mixture is heated through and creamy.
2. Serve:
   - Divide the coconut rice into bowls.
   - Top with diced mango and shredded coconut.
   - Garnish with fresh mint leaves if desired.

**Nutrition Info (per serving)**
- Calories: 320
- Protein: 5g
- Carbohydrates: 60g
- Fiber: 4g
- Sugars: 18g
- Total Fat: 9g
- Saturated Fat: 6g
- Cholesterol: 0mg
- Sodium: 30mg

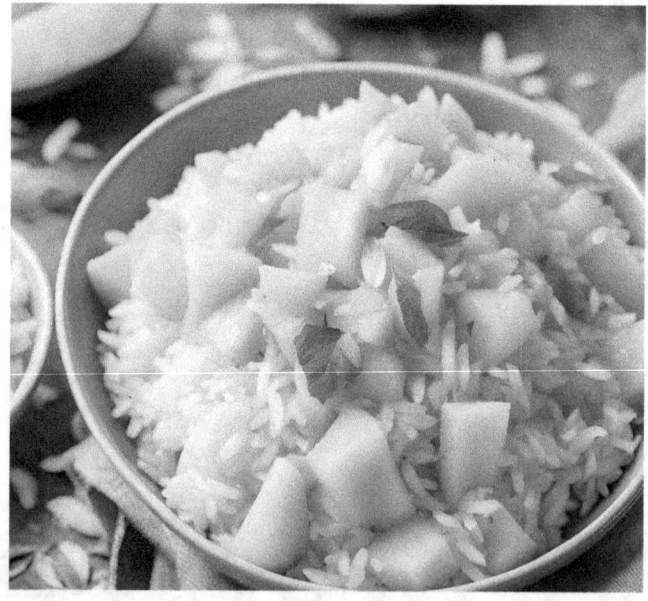

## 20. Savory Porridge

**Servings:** 2
**Cooking Time:** 15 minutes

**Ingredients**

- 1 cup rolled oats
- 2 cups vegetable broth
- 1/2 cup chopped spinach
- 1/4 cup diced tomatoes
- 1/4 cup diced bell peppers
- 1 tablespoon olive oil
- 1 teaspoon ground turmeric
- Freshly ground black pepper
- Fresh parsley (optional, for garnish)

**Instructions**

1. Cook the Oats:
   - In a medium saucepan, bring the vegetable broth to a boil.
   - Add the rolled oats, reduce the heat to low, and simmer for about 5 minutes, stirring occasionally, until the oats are tender and the mixture has thickened.
2. Add Vegetables and Spices:
   - Stir in the spinach, tomatoes, bell peppers, ground turmeric, and black pepper.
   - Cook for another 2-3 minutes until the vegetables are tender and well combined.
3. Serve:
   - Divide the savory porridge into bowls.
   - Garnish with fresh parsley if desired.

**Nutrition Info (per serving)**

- Calories: 210
- Protein: 6g
- Carbohydrates: 34g
- Fiber: 6g
- Sugars: 4g
- Total Fat: 6g
- Saturated Fat: 1g
- Cholesterol: 0mg
- Sodium: 360mg

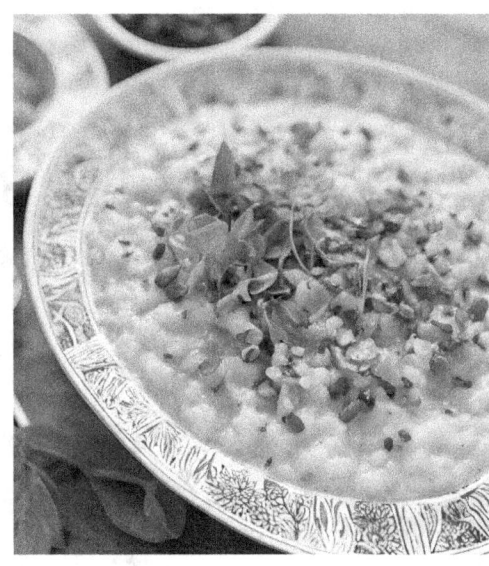

## 21. Stuffed Breakfast Peppers

**Servings:** 2
**Cooking Time:** 30 minutes

**Ingredients**
- 2 large bell peppers, halved and seeds removed
- 4 large eggs
- 1/4 cup diced tomatoes
- 1/4 cup chopped spinach
- 1/4 cup chopped onions
- 1/4 cup crumbled feta cheese
- 1 teaspoon dried oregano
- Freshly ground black pepper
- 1 tablespoon olive oil

**Instructions**
1. Preheat Oven:
   - Preheat your oven to 375°F (190°C).
2. Prepare the Filling:
   - In a bowl, whisk the eggs and stir in the diced tomatoes, chopped spinach, onions, dried oregano, and black pepper.
3. Stuff the Peppers:
   - Place the bell pepper halves in a baking dish.
   - Fill each pepper half with the egg mixture and top with crumbled feta cheese.
4. Bake:
   - Drizzle olive oil over the peppers.
   - Bake for 25-30 minutes, or until the eggs are set and the peppers are tender.
5. Serve:
   - Let cool for a few minutes before serving.

**Nutrition Info (per serving)**
- Calories: 250
- Protein: 14g
- Carbohydrates: 10g
- Fiber: 3g
- Sugars: 6g
- Total Fat: 18g
- Saturated Fat: 6g
- Cholesterol: 375mg
- Sodium: 250mg

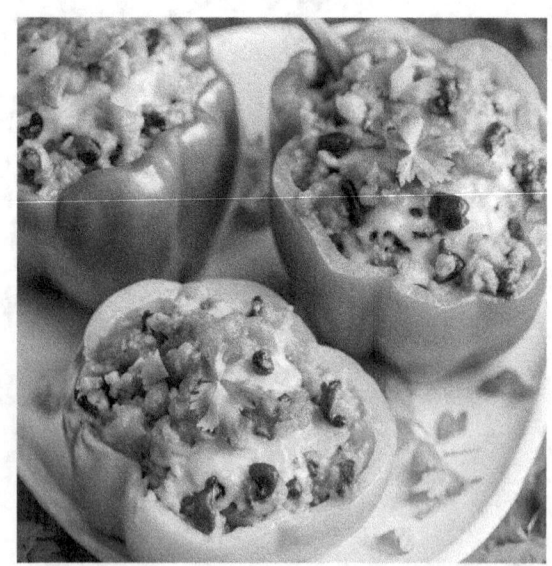

## 22. Apple-Cinnamon Oat Bake

**Servings:** 4
**Cooking Time:** 45 minutes

**Ingredients**
- 2 cups rolled oats
- 2 cups unsweetened almond milk (or any preferred non-dairy milk)
- 2 apples, peeled, cored, and diced
- 1/4 cup maple syrup
- 2 teaspoons ground cinnamon
- 1 teaspoon vanilla extract
- 1/4 cup chopped nuts (such as walnuts or pecans)
- 1 tablespoon chia seeds

**Instructions**
1. Preheat Oven:
   - Preheat your oven to 350°F (175°C).
2. Prepare the Oat Mixture:
   - In a large bowl, combine the rolled oats, almond milk, diced apples, maple syrup, ground cinnamon, vanilla extract, chopped nuts, and chia seeds. Mix well.
3. Bake:
   - Pour the mixture into a greased baking dish.
   - Bake for 35-40 minutes, or until the top is golden brown and the oats are set.
4. Serve:
   - Let cool slightly before cutting into portions.

**Nutrition Info (per serving)**
- Calories: 290
- Protein: 6g
- Carbohydrates: 50g
- Fiber: 7g
- Sugars: 18g
- Total Fat: 8g
- Saturated Fat: 0.5g
- Cholesterol: 0mg
- Sodium: 40mg

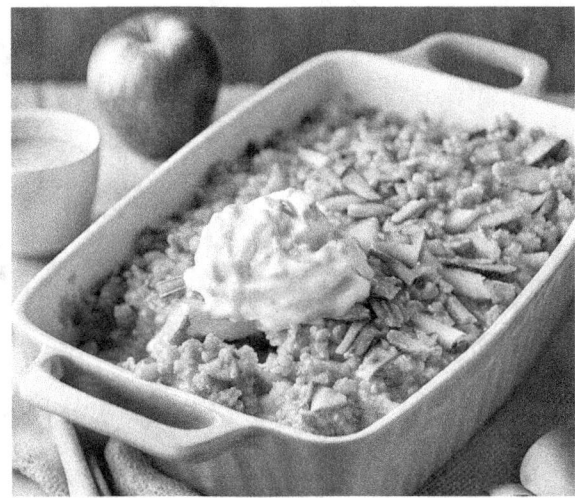

## 23. Almond Flour Waffles

**Servings:** 4
**Cooking Time:** 20 minutes

**Ingredients**
- 2 cups almond flour
- 3 large eggs
- 1/2 cup unsweetened almond milk (or any preferred non-dairy milk)
- 1 tablespoon coconut oil, melted
- 1 teaspoon vanilla extract
- 1 teaspoon baking powder
- Fresh fruit and nuts for topping

**Instructions**
1. Preheat Waffle Iron:
   - Preheat your waffle iron according to the manufacturer's instructions.
2. Prepare the Batter:
   - In a large bowl, whisk together the almond flour, eggs, almond milk, melted coconut oil, vanilla extract, and baking powder until smooth.
3. Cook the Waffles:
   - Pour the batter onto the preheated waffle iron and cook according to the manufacturer's instructions until the waffles are golden brown and cooked through.
4. Serve:
   - Top with fresh fruit and nuts.

**Nutrition Info (per serving)**
- Calories: 330
- Protein: 12g
- Carbohydrates: 12g
- Fiber: 5g
- Sugars: 3g
- Total Fat: 28g
- Saturated Fat: 4g
- Cholesterol: 110mg
- Sodium: 100mg

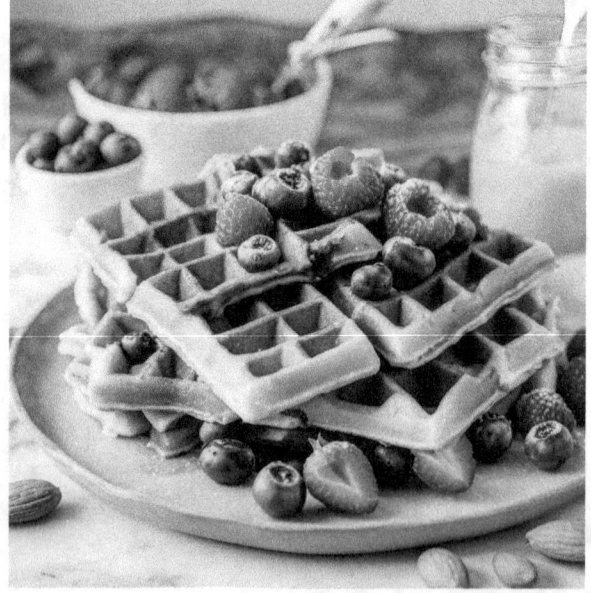

## 24. Zucchini and Onion Frittata

**Servings:** 4
**Cooking Time:** 30 minutes

**Ingredients**
- 6 large eggs
- 2 medium zucchinis, sliced
- 1 small onion, chopped
- 1/4 cup grated Parmesan cheese
- 1 tablespoon olive oil
- 1 teaspoon dried thyme
- Freshly ground black pepper

**Instructions**

1. Preheat Oven:
   - Preheat your oven to 375°F (190°C).
2. Cook the Vegetables:
   - In an oven-safe skillet, heat the olive oil over medium heat.
   - Add the chopped onion and cook for 3-4 minutes until softened.
   - Add the sliced zucchini and cook for another 5-7 minutes until tender.
3. Prepare the Egg Mixture:
   - In a bowl, whisk the eggs and stir in the grated Parmesan cheese, dried thyme, and black pepper.
4. Combine and Bake:
   - Pour the egg mixture over the vegetables in the skillet.
   - Cook on the stovetop for 2-3 minutes until the edges start to set.
   - Transfer the skillet to the preheated oven and bake for 15-20 minutes, or until the frittata is fully set and golden brown on top.
5. Serve:
   - Let cool slightly before slicing and serving.

**Nutrition Info (per serving)**
- Calories: 200
- Protein: 13g
- Carbohydrates: 5g
- Fiber: 1g
- Sugars: 3g
- Total Fat: 14g
- Saturated Fat: 4g
- Cholesterol: 220mg
- Sodium: 180mg

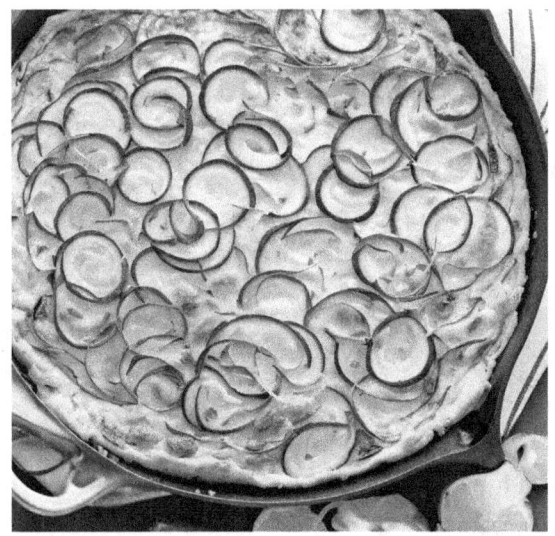

## 25. Shakshuka

**Servings: 4**
**Cooking Time: 30 minutes**
**Ingredients**

- 2 tablespoons olive oil
- 1 medium onion, chopped
- 1 red bell pepper, diced
- 3 cloves garlic, minced
- 1 teaspoon ground cumin
- 1 teaspoon ground paprika
- 1/4 teaspoon cayenne pepper
- 1 can (28 ounces) diced tomatoes
- 4 large eggs
- Freshly ground black pepper
- Fresh cilantro or parsley (optional, for garnish)

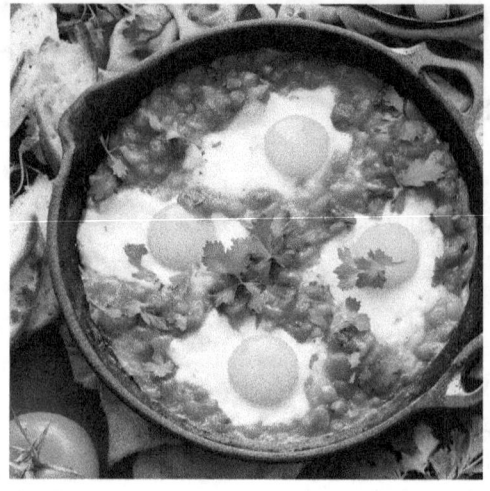

**Instructions**

1. Cook the Vegetables:
   - In a large skillet, heat the olive oil over medium heat.
   - Add the chopped onion and cook for 3-4 minutes until softened.
   - Add the diced bell pepper and cook for another 5 minutes.
   - Stir in the minced garlic, ground cumin, ground paprika, and cayenne pepper. Cook for 1-2 minutes until fragrant.
2. Add Tomatoes:
   - Pour in the diced tomatoes with their juice.
   - Simmer for 10-15 minutes, stirring occasionally, until the sauce thickens slightly.
3. Poach the Eggs:
   - Make four small wells in the sauce and crack an egg into each well.
   - Cover the skillet and cook for 5-7 minutes, or until the eggs are set to your liking.
4. Serve:
   - Season with freshly ground black pepper.
   - Garnish with fresh cilantro or parsley if desired.

**Nutrition Info (per serving)**

- Calories: 180
- Protein: 8g
- Carbohydrates: 14g
- Fiber: 4g
- Sugars: 8g
- Total Fat: 10g
- Saturated Fat: 2g
- Cholesterol: 185mg
- Sodium: 340mg

# Fish and Seafood Recipes

**1. Grilled Salmon with Dill Yogurt Sauce**
**Servings: 4**
**Cooking Time: 20 minutes**
**Ingredients**
- 4 salmon fillets (about 6 ounces each)
- 2 tablespoons olive oil
- 1 teaspoon dried dill
- 1 cup plain Greek yogurt
- 1 tablespoon fresh dill, chopped
- 1 tablespoon lemon juice
- 1 garlic clove, minced
- Freshly ground black pepper
- Lemon wedges (for serving)

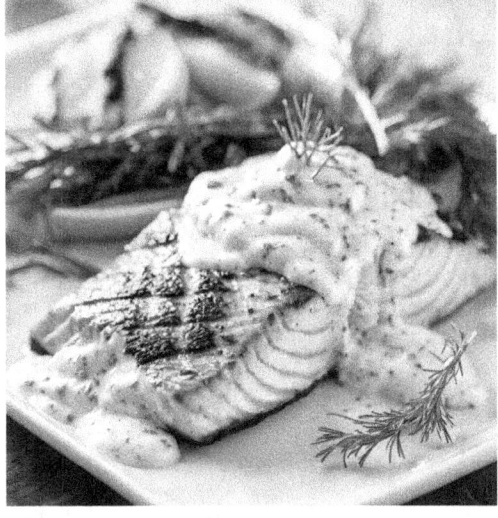

**Instructions**
1. Prepare the Salmon:
   - Preheat the grill to medium-high heat.
   - Brush the salmon fillets with olive oil and sprinkle with dried dill and black pepper.
2. Grill the Salmon:
   - Place the salmon fillets on the grill and cook for 4-5 minutes per side, or until the fish flakes easily with a fork.
3. Prepare the Dill Yogurt Sauce:
   - In a small bowl, mix the Greek yogurt, fresh dill, lemon juice, minced garlic, and freshly ground black pepper.
4. Serve:
   - Serve the grilled salmon with a generous dollop of dill yogurt sauce and lemon wedges on the side.

**Nutrition Info (per serving)**
- Calories: 350
- Protein: 35g
- Carbohydrates: 4g
- Fiber: 0g
- Sugars: 3g
- Total Fat: 22g
- Saturated Fat: 4g
- Cholesterol: 95mg
- Sodium: 80mg

## 2. Baked Cod with Lemon and Capers

**Servings:** 4
**Cooking Time:** 25 minutes

**Ingredients**

- 4 cod fillets (about 6 ounces each)
- 2 tablespoons olive oil
- 1/4 cup lemon juice
- 2 tablespoons capers, drained
- 1 teaspoon dried oregano
- Freshly ground black pepper
- Fresh parsley (optional, for garnish)

**Instructions**

1. Preheat Oven:
   - Preheat your oven to 375°F (190°C).
2. Prepare the Cod:
   - Place the cod fillets in a baking dish.
   - Drizzle with olive oil and lemon juice.
   - Sprinkle with capers, dried oregano, and freshly ground black pepper.
3. Bake:
   - Bake for 20-25 minutes, or until the fish flakes easily with a fork.
4. Serve:
   - Garnish with fresh parsley if desired.

**Nutrition Info (per serving)**

- Calories: 220
- Protein: 28g
- Carbohydrates: 2g
- Fiber: 0g
- Sugars: 0g
- Total Fat: 10g
- Saturated Fat: 2g
- Cholesterol: 75mg
- Sodium: 290mg

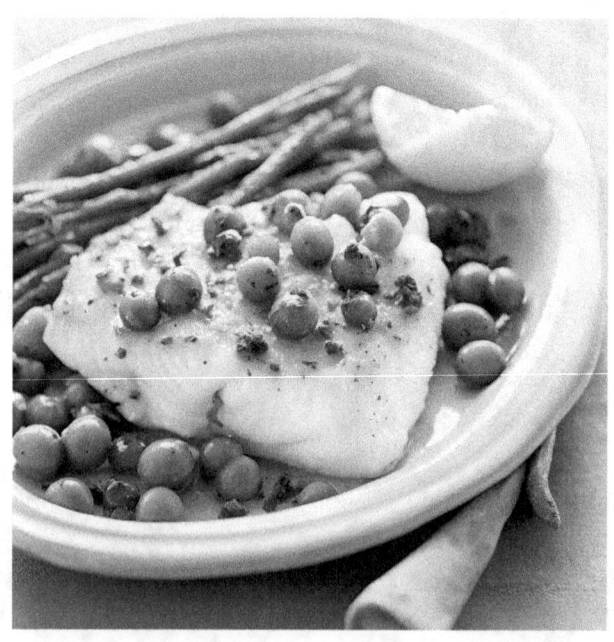

## 3. Shrimp and Avocado Salad

**Servings:** 4
**Cooking Time:** 15 minutes

**Ingredients**

- 1 pound cooked shrimp, peeled and deveined
- 2 avocados, diced
- 1 cup cherry tomatoes, halved
- 1/4 cup red onion, finely chopped
- 2 tablespoons fresh lime juice
- 2 tablespoons olive oil
- 1 teaspoon ground cumin
- Freshly ground black pepper
- Fresh cilantro (optional, for garnish)

**Instructions**

1. Prepare the Salad:
    - In a large bowl, combine the cooked shrimp, diced avocados, cherry tomatoes, and red onion.
2. Prepare the Dressing:
    - In a small bowl, whisk together the lime juice, olive oil, ground cumin, and freshly ground black pepper.
3. Toss the Salad:
    - Pour the dressing over the shrimp and avocado mixture and toss gently to combine.
4. Serve:
    - Garnish with fresh cilantro if desired.

**Nutrition Info (per serving)**

- Calories: 300
- Protein: 22g
- Carbohydrates: 10g
- Fiber: 7g
- Sugars: 2g
- Total Fat: 20g
- Saturated Fat: 3g
- Cholesterol: 170mg
- Sodium: 320mg

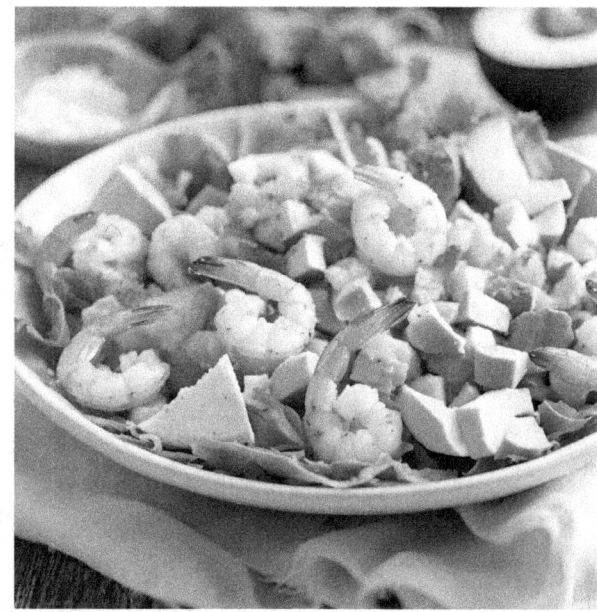

## 4. Herb-Crusted Tilapia

**Servings:** 4
**Cooking Time:** 20 minutes

**Ingredients**

- 4 tilapia fillets (about 6 ounces each)
- 1/2 cup whole wheat bread crumbs
- 1/4 cup grated Parmesan cheese
- 2 tablespoons fresh parsley, chopped
- 1 tablespoon fresh thyme, chopped
- 1 tablespoon olive oil
- Freshly ground black pepper
- Lemon wedges (for serving)

**Instructions**

1. Preheat Oven:
   - Preheat your oven to 400°F (200°C).
2. Prepare the Herb Crust:
   - In a bowl, combine the whole wheat bread crumbs, grated Parmesan cheese, chopped parsley, chopped thyme, and freshly ground black pepper.
   - Add the olive oil and mix until the bread crumbs are evenly coated.
3. Coat the Tilapia:
   - Place the tilapia fillets on a baking sheet lined with parchment paper.
   - Press the herb crumb mixture onto the top of each fillet.
4. Bake:
   - Bake for 15-20 minutes, or until the fish flakes easily with a fork and the crust is golden brown.
5. Serve:
   - Serve with lemon wedges.

**Nutrition Info (per serving)**

- Calories: 280
- Protein: 30g
- Carbohydrates: 10g
- Fiber: 2g
- Sugars: 1g
- Total Fat: 14g
- Saturated Fat: 3g
- Cholesterol: 70mg
- Sodium: 180mg

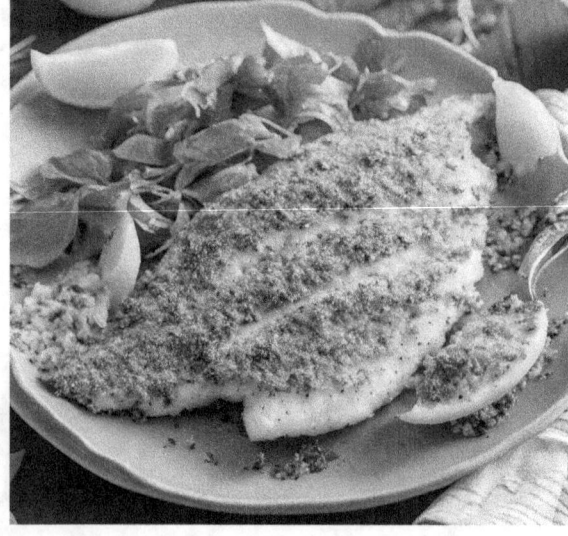

## 5. Scallop Stir-Fry

**Servings: 4**
**Cooking Time: 20 minutes**
**Ingredients**

- 1 pound sea scallops
- 2 tablespoons olive oil
- 1 red bell pepper, sliced
- 1 yellow bell pepper, sliced
- 1 cup snow peas
- 1 cup broccoli florets
- 2 cloves garlic, minced
- 2 tablespoons low-sodium soy sauce
- 1 tablespoon fresh ginger, grated
- 1 tablespoon sesame oil
- Freshly ground black pepper
- Fresh cilantro (optional, for garnish)

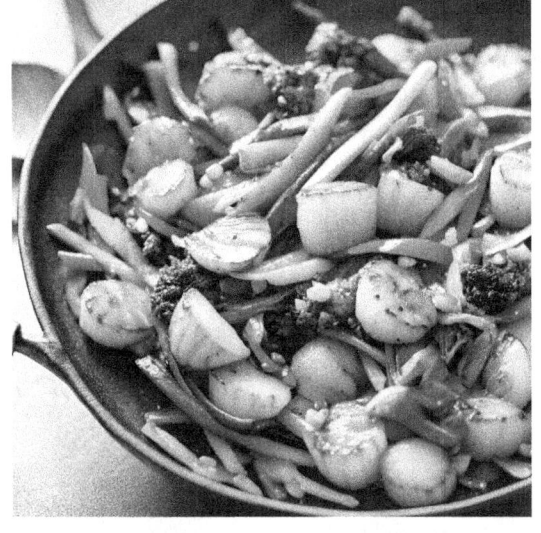

**Instructions**

1. Prepare the Vegetables:
   - Heat the olive oil in a large skillet or wok over medium-high heat.
   - Add the red bell pepper, yellow bell pepper, snow peas, and broccoli florets. Stir-fry for 5-7 minutes until the vegetables are tender-crisp.
2. Cook the Scallops:
   - Push the vegetables to the side of the skillet and add the scallops.
   - Cook for 2-3 minutes on each side until the scallops are opaque and cooked through.
3. Add Flavorings:
   - Stir in the minced garlic, grated ginger, low-sodium soy sauce, sesame oil, and freshly ground black pepper.
   - Toss everything together until well combined and heated through.
4. Serve:
   - Garnish with fresh cilantro if desired.

**Nutrition Info (per serving)**

- Calories: 240
- Protein: 25g
- Carbohydrates: 10g
- Fiber: 3g
- Sugars: 4g
- Total Fat: 10g
- Saturated Fat: 1.5g
- Cholesterol: 35mg
- Sodium: 450mg

## 6. Fish Tacos with Cabbage Slaw

**Servings:** 4
**Cooking Time:** 25 minutes

**Ingredients**

- 1 pound white fish fillets (such as cod or tilapia)
- 2 tablespoons olive oil
- 1 teaspoon ground cumin
- 1 teaspoon paprika
- 1/4 teaspoon cayenne pepper
- 8 small corn tortillas
- 2 cups shredded cabbage
- 1/4 cup chopped cilantro
- 1/4 cup plain Greek yogurt
- 1 tablespoon lime juice
- Freshly ground black pepper
- Lime wedges (for serving)

**Instructions**

1. Prepare the Fish:
    - Preheat the oven to 400°F (200°C).
    - Place the fish fillets on a baking sheet and drizzle with olive oil.
    - Sprinkle with ground cumin, paprika, cayenne pepper, and freshly ground black pepper.
    - Bake for 15-20 minutes, or until the fish flakes easily with a fork.
2. Prepare the Cabbage Slaw:
    - In a bowl, combine the shredded cabbage, chopped cilantro, Greek yogurt, lime juice, and freshly ground black pepper. Mix well.
3. Assemble the Tacos:
    - Warm the corn tortillas in a skillet or microwave.
    - Break the fish into chunks and distribute evenly among the tortillas.
    - Top with cabbage slaw.
4. Serve:
    - Serve with lime wedges on the side.

**Nutrition Info (per serving)**

- Calories: 310
- Protein: 28g
- Carbohydrates: 24g
- Fiber: 6g
- Sugars: 3g
- Total Fat: 12g
- Saturated Fat: 2g
- Cholesterol: 60mg
- Sodium: 120mg

## 7. Crab Stuffed Mushrooms

**Servings:** 4
**Cooking Time:** 30 minutes

**Ingredients**
- 12 large mushroom caps
- 1 cup cooked crab meat
- 1/4 cup whole wheat bread crumbs
- 1/4 cup grated Parmesan cheese
- 1/4 cup chopped green onions
- 1 tablespoon olive oil
- 1 tablespoon fresh lemon juice
- 1 teaspoon dried dill
- Freshly ground black pepper

**Instructions**

1. Preheat Oven:
   - Preheat your oven to 375°F (190°C).
2. Prepare the Filling:
   - In a bowl, combine the crab meat, bread crumbs, Parmesan cheese, chopped green onions, olive oil, lemon juice, dried dill, and freshly ground black pepper.
3. Stuff the Mushrooms:
   - Place the mushroom caps on a baking sheet.
   - Fill each mushroom cap with the crab mixture.
4. Bake:
   - Bake for 20-25 minutes, or until the mushrooms are tender and the filling is golden brown.
5. Serve:
   - Serve warm.

**Nutrition Info (per serving)**
- Calories: 180
- Protein: 15g
- Carbohydrates: 12g
- Fiber: 2g
- Sugars: 3g
- Total Fat: 8g
- Saturated Fat: 2g
- Cholesterol: 45mg
- Sodium: 290mg

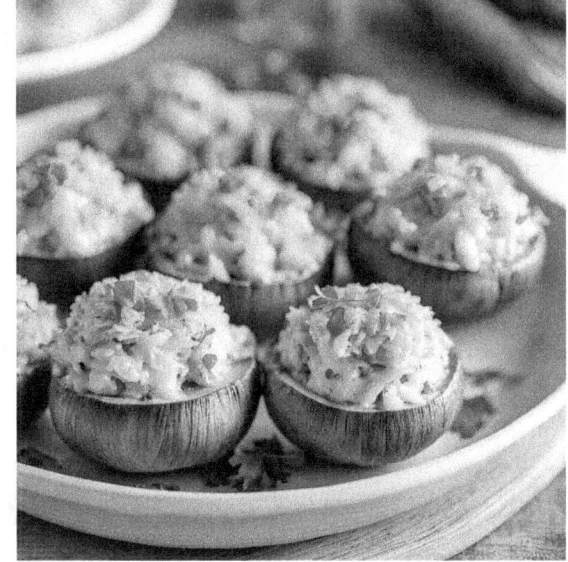

## 8. Tuna Nicoise Salad

**Servings:** 4
**Cooking Time:** 20 minutes

**Ingredients**

- 2 cans (6 ounces each) tuna in water, drained
- 8 ounces green beans, trimmed and blanched
- 4 small red potatoes, cooked and quartered
- 2 hard-boiled eggs, quartered
- 1 cup cherry tomatoes, halved
- 1/4 cup black olives
- 1/4 cup chopped red onion
- 4 cups mixed salad greens
- 1/4 cup olive oil
- 2 tablespoons red wine vinegar
- 1 teaspoon Dijon mustard
- Freshly ground black pepper

**Instructions**

1. Prepare the Dressing:
   - In a small bowl, whisk together the olive oil, red wine vinegar, Dijon mustard, and freshly ground black pepper.
2. Assemble the Salad:
   - On a large platter or individual plates, arrange the salad greens.
   - Top with green beans, red potatoes, hard-boiled eggs, cherry tomatoes, black olives, and chopped red onion.
   - Flake the tuna over the salad.
3. Serve:
   - Drizzle the dressing over the salad and serve immediately.

**Nutrition Info (per serving)**

- Calories: 330
- Protein: 22g
- Carbohydrates: 18g
- Fiber: 4g
- Sugars: 3g
- Total Fat: 20g
- Saturated Fat: 3g
- Cholesterol: 140mg
- Sodium: 350mg

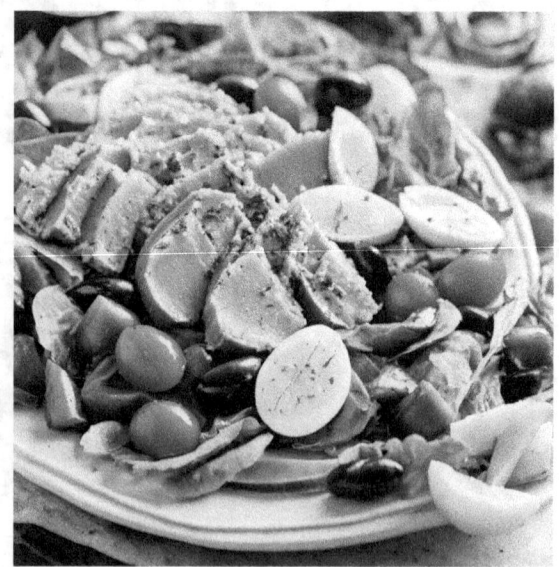

## 9. Lemon Garlic Shrimp

**Servings:** 4
**Cooking Time:** 15 minutes

**Ingredients**

- 1 pound large shrimp, peeled and deveined
- 2 tablespoons olive oil
- 3 cloves garlic, minced
- 1 tablespoon fresh lemon juice
- 1 teaspoon lemon zest
- 1/4 cup chopped fresh parsley
- Freshly ground black pepper
- Lemon wedges (for serving)

**Instructions**

1. Cook the Shrimp:
   - In a large skillet, heat the olive oil over medium heat.
   - Add the minced garlic and cook for 1-2 minutes until fragrant.
   - Add the shrimp and cook for 3-4 minutes on each side until pink and opaque.
2. Add Lemon and Parsley:
   - Stir in the lemon juice, lemon zest, and freshly ground black pepper.
   - Remove from heat and stir in the chopped parsley.
3. Serve:
   - Serve with lemon wedges on the side.

**Nutrition Info (per serving)**

- Calories: 180
- Protein: 24g
- Carbohydrates: 2g
- Fiber: 0g
- Sugars: 0g
- Total Fat: 8g
- Saturated Fat: 1g
- Cholesterol: 190mg
- Sodium: 220mg

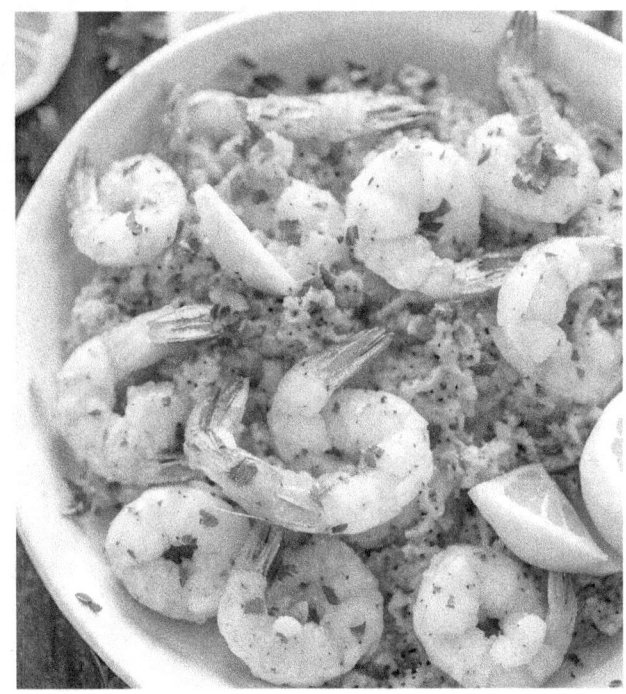

## 10. Mackerel Pate

**Servings:** 4
**Cooking Time:** 10 minutes
**Ingredients**

- 8 ounces smoked mackerel, skin removed
- 1/2 cup plain Greek yogurt
- 1 tablespoon lemon juice
- 1 teaspoon lemon zest
- 1 tablespoon chopped fresh dill
- Freshly ground black pepper
- Whole grain crackers or vegetable sticks (for serving)

**Instructions**

1. Prepare the Pate:
    - In a food processor, combine the smoked mackerel, Greek yogurt, lemon juice, lemon zest, chopped dill, and freshly ground black pepper.
    - Process until smooth and well combined.
2. Serve:
    - Transfer the pate to a serving bowl.
    - Serve with whole grain crackers or vegetable sticks.

**Nutrition Info (per serving)**

- Calories: 200
- Protein: 18g
- Carbohydrates: 4g
- Fiber: 0g
- Sugars: 2g
- Total Fat: 12g
- Saturated Fat: 2g
- Cholesterol: 50mg
- Sodium: 400mg

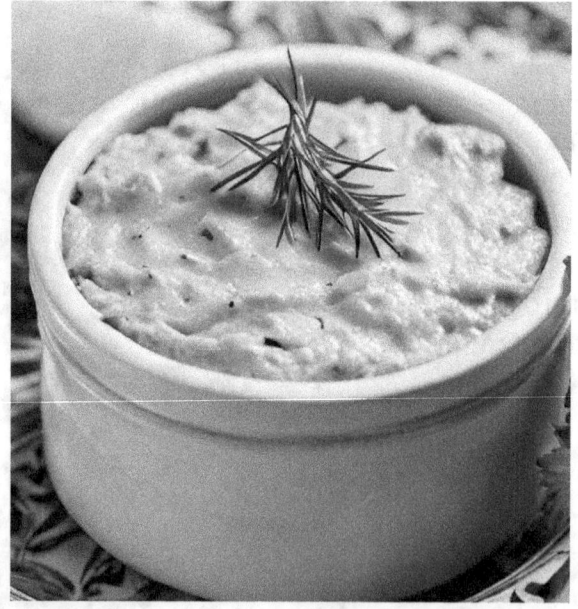

## 11. Baked Trout with Almonds

**Servings:** 4
**Cooking Time:** 25 minutes

**Ingredients**

- 4 trout fillets (about 6 ounces each)
- 1/4 cup sliced almonds
- 2 tablespoons olive oil
- 1 lemon, thinly sliced
- 1 teaspoon dried thyme
- Freshly ground black pepper
- Fresh parsley (optional, for garnish)

**Instructions**

1. Preheat Oven:
   - Preheat your oven to 375°F (190°C).
2. Prepare the Trout:
   - Place the trout fillets on a baking sheet lined with parchment paper.
   - Drizzle with olive oil and sprinkle with dried thyme and freshly ground black pepper.
   - Top with lemon slices and sliced almonds.
3. Bake:
   - Bake for 20-25 minutes, or until the trout flakes easily with a fork and the almonds are golden brown.
4. Serve:
   - Garnish with fresh parsley if desired.

**Nutrition Info (per serving)**

- Calories: 310
- Protein: 28g
- Carbohydrates: 4g
- Fiber: 2g
- Sugars: 1g
- Total Fat: 20g
- Saturated Fat: 3g
- Cholesterol: 80mg
- Sodium: 80mg

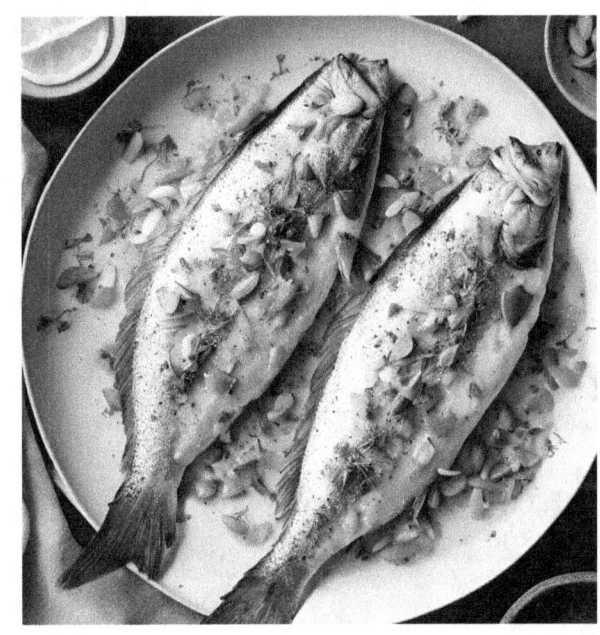

## 12. Haddock in Parchment

**Servings:** 4
**Cooking Time:** 30 minutes

**Ingredients**

- 4 haddock fillets (about 6 ounces each)
- 2 cups thinly sliced zucchini
- 1 cup cherry tomatoes, halved
- 1 small red onion, thinly sliced
- 1 lemon, thinly sliced
- 2 tablespoons olive oil
- 1 teaspoon dried oregano
- Freshly ground black pepper
- Fresh parsley (optional, for garnish)
- Parchment paper

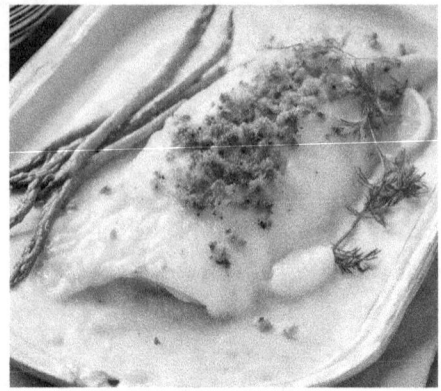

**Instructions**

1. Preheat Oven:
   - Preheat your oven to 400°F (200°C).
2. Prepare the Vegetables:
   - In a bowl, toss the zucchini, cherry tomatoes, and red onion with olive oil, dried oregano, and freshly ground black pepper.
3. Prepare the Parchment Packets:
   - Cut four large pieces of parchment paper.
   - Place a haddock fillet in the center of each piece of parchment.
   - Divide the vegetable mixture evenly over the fillets.
   - Top with lemon slices.
   - Fold the parchment paper over the fish and vegetables, sealing the edges to form packets.
4. Bake:
   - Place the parchment packets on a baking sheet and bake for 20-25 minutes, or until the fish is cooked through and flakes easily with a fork.
5. Serve:
   - Carefully open the packets and transfer the fish and vegetables to plates.
   - Garnish with fresh parsley if desired.

**Nutrition Info (per serving)**

- Calories: 260   Protein: 30g   Carbohydrates: 10g   Fiber: 3g
- Sugars: 5g
- Total Fat: 12g
- Saturated Fat: 2g
- Cholesterol: 80mg
- Sodium: 100mg

## 13. Scallop and Pea Risotto

**Servings:** 4
**Cooking Time:** 35 minutes

**Ingredients**
- 1 pound sea scallops
- 1 cup arborio rice
- 1 small onion, finely chopped
- 3 cloves garlic, minced
- 4 cups low-sodium chicken or vegetable broth
- 1 cup frozen peas, thawed
- 1/4 cup grated Parmesan cheese
- 2 tablespoons olive oil
- 1 tablespoon fresh lemon juice
- Freshly ground black pepper
- Fresh parsley (optional, for garnish)

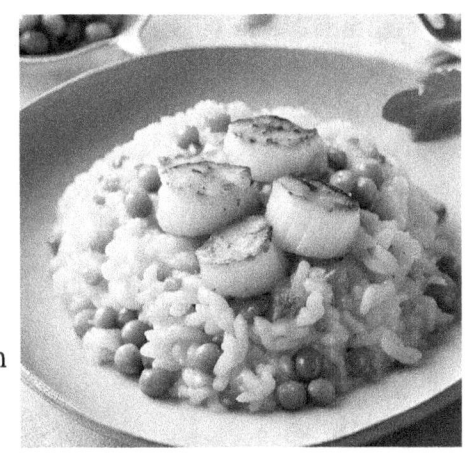

**Instructions**
1. Prepare the Broth:
   - In a saucepan, heat the broth and keep it warm over low heat.
2. Cook the Scallops:
   - In a large skillet, heat 1 tablespoon of olive oil over medium-high heat.
   - Add the scallops and cook for 2-3 minutes on each side until they are opaque and slightly golden.
   - Remove the scallops from the skillet and set aside.
3. Prepare the Risotto:
   - In the same skillet, add the remaining olive oil and the chopped onion. Cook for 3-4 minutes until the onion is softened.
   - Add the minced garlic and arborio rice. Cook for 2 minutes, stirring constantly.
4. Add Broth Gradually:
   - Add one ladleful of warm broth to the rice mixture and stir until the liquid is absorbed.
   - Continue adding the broth one ladleful at a time, stirring frequently, until the rice is creamy and tender, about 18-20 minutes.
5. Finish the Risotto:
   - Stir in the thawed peas, grated Parmesan cheese, fresh lemon juice, and freshly ground black pepper.
   - Gently fold in the cooked scallops.
6. Serve:
   - Divide the risotto among plates and garnish with fresh parsley if desired.

**Nutrition Info (per serving)**
- Calories: 390   Protein: 26g   Carbohydrates: 45g   Fiber: 4g
- Sugars: 4g   Total Fat: 12g   Saturated Fat: 3g   Cholesterol: 45mg   Sodium: 400mg

## 14. Grilled Tuna Steaks

**Servings:** 4
**Cooking Time:** 15 minutes

**Ingredients**

- 4 tuna steaks (about 6 ounces each)
- 2 tablespoons olive oil
- 1 tablespoon fresh lemon juice
- 1 teaspoon dried oregano
- Freshly ground black pepper
- Lemon wedges (for serving)

**Instructions**

1. Prepare the Tuna:
   - Preheat the grill to medium-high heat.
   - Brush the tuna steaks with olive oil and drizzle with lemon juice.
   - Sprinkle with dried oregano and freshly ground black pepper.
2. Grill the Tuna:
   - Place the tuna steaks on the grill and cook for 3-4 minutes on each side for medium-rare, or until cooked to your desired level of doneness.
3. Serve:
   - Serve the grilled tuna steaks with lemon wedges on the side.

**Nutrition Info (per serving)**

- Calories: 250
- Protein: 35g
- Carbohydrates: 1g
- Fiber: 0g
- Sugars: 0g
- Total Fat: 12g
- Saturated Fat: 2g
- Cholesterol: 60mg
- Sodium: 70mg

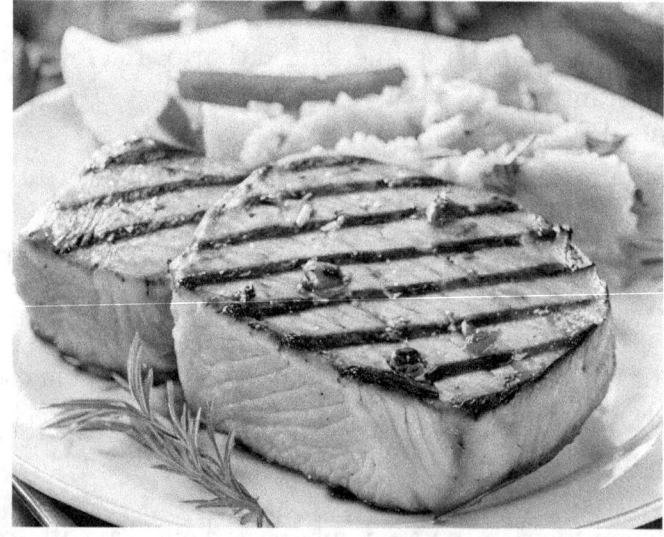

## 15. Sardines on Toast

**Servings:** 4
**Cooking Time:** 10 minutes

**Ingredients**

- 8 sardines, cleaned and filleted
- 4 slices of whole grain bread
- 1 tablespoon olive oil
- 1 lemon, thinly sliced
- 1 garlic clove, minced
- 1 tablespoon fresh parsley, chopped
- Freshly ground black pepper

**Instructions**

1. Prepare the Bread:
   - Toast the slices of whole grain bread to your desired level of crispiness.
2. Cook the Sardines:
   - In a skillet, heat the olive oil over medium heat.
   - Add the minced garlic and cook for 1-2 minutes until fragrant.
   - Add the sardine fillets and lemon slices. Cook for 2-3 minutes on each side until the sardines are cooked through and the lemon slices are slightly caramelized.
3. Assemble the Toast:
   - Place the cooked sardines on the toasted bread.
   - Top with caramelized lemon slices and sprinkle with freshly ground black pepper and chopped parsley.
4. Serve:
   - Serve immediately.

**Nutrition Info (per serving)**

- Calories: 290
- Protein: 20g
- Carbohydrates: 18g
- Fiber: 4g
- Sugars: 1g
- Total Fat: 16g
- Saturated Fat: 3g
- Cholesterol: 45mg
- Sodium: 280mg

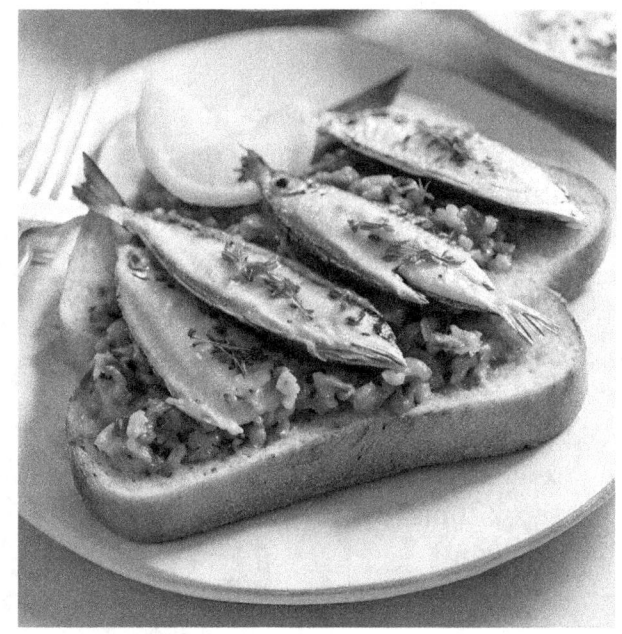

## 16. Mussels in Tomato Broth

**Servings:** 4
**Cooking Time:** 20 minutes

**Ingredients**
- 2 pounds fresh mussels, cleaned and debearded
- 2 tablespoons olive oil
- 1 onion, finely chopped
- 3 cloves garlic, minced
- 1 can (14.5 ounces) diced tomatoes
- 1 cup low-sodium vegetable broth
- 1/2 cup white wine (optional)
- 1 teaspoon dried oregano
- Freshly ground black pepper
- Fresh parsley (optional, for garnish)

**Instructions**

1. Prepare the Broth:
   - In a large pot, heat the olive oil over medium heat.
   - Add the onion and cook for 3-4 minutes until softened.
   - Add the minced garlic and cook for another 1-2 minutes.
2. Add Tomatoes and Seasoning:
   - Stir in the diced tomatoes, vegetable broth, white wine (if using), dried oregano, and freshly ground black pepper.
   - Bring to a simmer and cook for 5 minutes.
3. Cook the Mussels:
   - Add the mussels to the pot, cover, and cook for 5-7 minutes, or until the mussels have opened. Discard any mussels that do not open.
4. Serve:
   - Divide the mussels and tomato broth among bowls.
   - Garnish with fresh parsley if desired.

**Nutrition Info (per serving)**
- Calories: 220
- Protein: 18g
- Carbohydrates: 12g
- Fiber: 2g
- Sugars: 5g
- Total Fat: 9g
- Saturated Fat: 1.5g
- Cholesterol: 40mg
- Sodium: 480mg

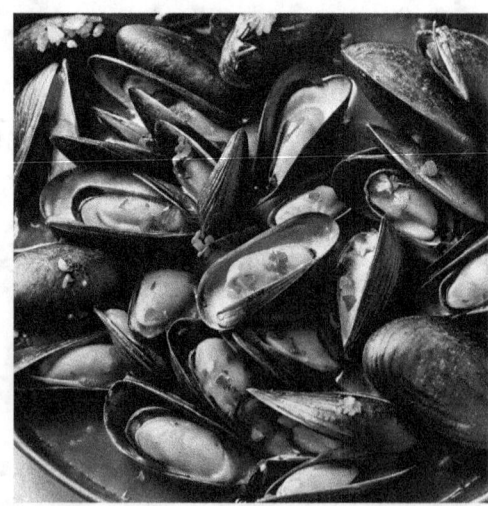

## 17. Ceviche

**Servings:** 4
**Cooking Time:** 15 minutes (plus 30 minutes for marinating)
**Ingredients**
- 1 pound white fish fillets (such as tilapia or snapper), diced
- 1 cup fresh lime juice
- 1/2 cup diced red onion
- 1 jalapeño, seeded and finely chopped
- 1 cup diced tomatoes
- 1 avocado, diced
- 1/4 cup chopped fresh cilantro
- Freshly ground black pepper
- 1 tablespoon olive oil
- Lettuce leaves (for serving)

**Instructions**
1. Marinate the Fish:
   - In a large glass bowl, combine the diced fish and lime juice. Ensure the fish is fully submerged.
   - Cover and refrigerate for 30 minutes, or until the fish is opaque and "cooked" by the lime juice.
2. Combine Ingredients:
   - Drain the fish, discarding the lime juice.
   - Add the diced red onion, jalapeño, tomatoes, avocado, fresh cilantro, and freshly ground black pepper.
   - Drizzle with olive oil and toss gently to combine.
3. Serve:
   - Serve the ceviche on lettuce leaves.

**Nutrition Info (per serving)**
- Calories: 220
- Protein: 22g
- Carbohydrates: 10g
- Fiber: 5g
- Sugars: 2g
- Total Fat: 10g
- Saturated Fat: 1.5g
- Cholesterol: 55mg
- Sodium: 80mg

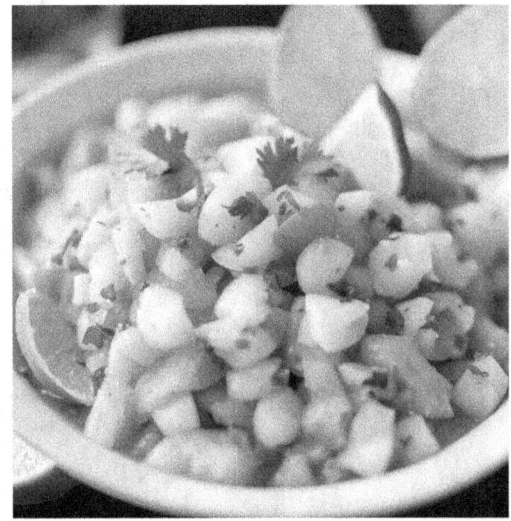

## 18. Sea Bass with Mango Salsa

**Servings:** 4
**Cooking Time:** 20 minutes

**Ingredients**
- 4 sea bass fillets (about 6 ounces each)
- 2 tablespoons olive oil
- 1 teaspoon ground cumin
- Freshly ground black pepper
- 1 mango, peeled and diced
- 1/2 red bell pepper, diced
- 1/4 red onion, finely chopped
- 1 tablespoon fresh lime juice
- 1 tablespoon chopped fresh cilantro

**Instructions**
1. Prepare the Sea Bass:
   - Preheat the oven to 400°F (200°C).
   - Brush the sea bass fillets with olive oil and sprinkle with ground cumin and freshly ground black pepper.
2. Bake the Sea Bass:
   - Place the fillets on a baking sheet lined with parchment paper.
   - Bake for 12-15 minutes, or until the fish flakes easily with a fork.
3. Prepare the Mango Salsa:
   - In a bowl, combine the diced mango, red bell pepper, red onion, lime juice, and chopped cilantro. Mix well.
4. Serve:
   - Top the baked sea bass with mango salsa.

**Nutrition Info (per serving)**
- Calories: 290
- Protein: 28g
- Carbohydrates: 12g
- Fiber: 2g
- Sugars: 8g
- Total Fat: 14g
- Saturated Fat: 2.5g
- Cholesterol: 70mg
- Sodium: 90mg

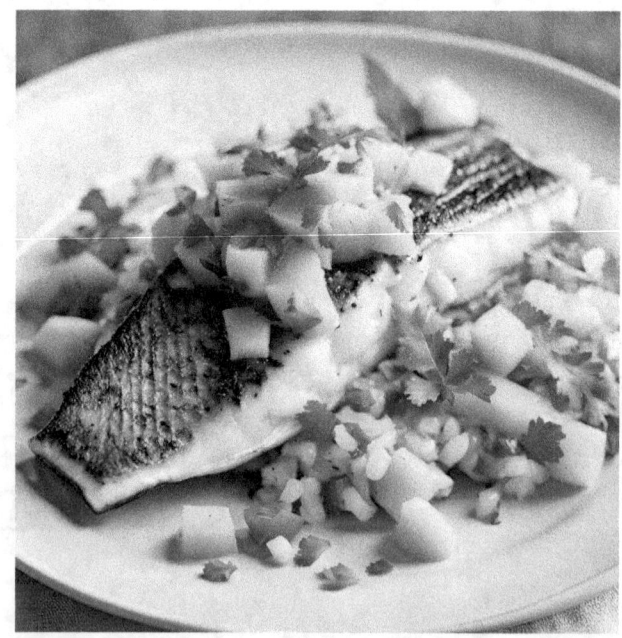

## 19. Garlic Butter Scallops

**Servings:** 4
**Cooking Time:** 15 minutes

**Ingredients**

- 1 pound sea scallops
- 2 tablespoons unsalted butter
- 2 tablespoons olive oil
- 3 cloves garlic, minced
- 1 tablespoon fresh lemon juice
- 1 teaspoon lemon zest
- Freshly ground black pepper
- Fresh parsley (optional, for garnish)

**Instructions**

1. Cook the Scallops:
   - In a large skillet, heat the olive oil over medium-high heat.
   - Add the scallops and cook for 2-3 minutes on each side until they are golden brown and opaque.
   - Remove the scallops from the skillet and set aside.
2. Prepare the Garlic Butter:
   - In the same skillet, reduce the heat to medium and add the butter.
   - Once melted, add the minced garlic and cook for 1-2 minutes until fragrant.
   - Stir in the lemon juice and lemon zest.
3. Combine and Serve:
   - Return the scallops to the skillet and toss to coat with the garlic butter.
   - Garnish with freshly ground black pepper and parsley if desired.

**Nutrition Info (per serving)**

- Calories: 240
- Protein: 24g
- Carbohydrates: 2g
- Fiber: 0g
- Sugars: 0g
- Total Fat: 14g
- Saturated Fat: 5g
- Cholesterol: 60mg
- Sodium: 270mg

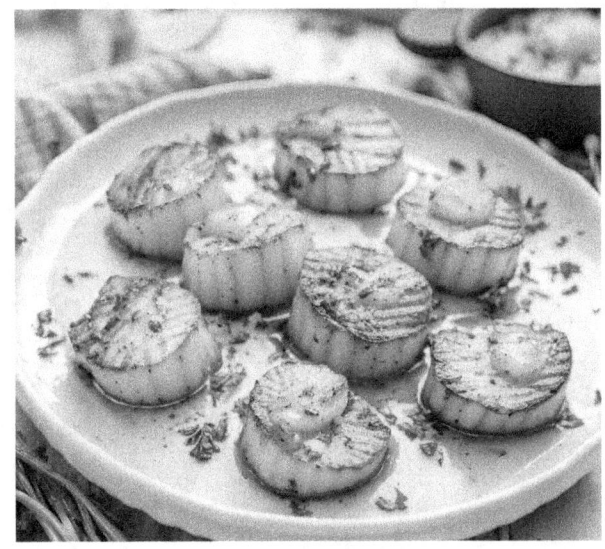

## 20. Parmesan Crusted Halibut

**Servings:** 4
**Cooking Time:** 25 minutes

**Ingredients**
- 4 halibut fillets (about 6 ounces each)
- 1/2 cup grated Parmesan cheese
- 1/2 cup whole wheat bread crumbs
- 2 tablespoons olive oil
- 1 teaspoon dried basil
- Freshly ground black pepper
- Lemon wedges (for serving)

**Instructions**
1. Preheat Oven:
   - Preheat your oven to 400°F (200°C).
2. Prepare the Crust:
   - In a bowl, combine the grated Parmesan cheese, whole wheat bread crumbs, dried basil, and freshly ground black pepper.
   - Add the olive oil and mix until the crumbs are evenly coated.
3. Coat the Halibut:
   - Place the halibut fillets on a baking sheet lined with parchment paper.
   - Press the Parmesan crumb mixture onto the top of each fillet.
4. Bake:
   - Bake for 15-20 minutes, or until the fish flakes easily with a fork and the crust is golden brown.
5. Serve:
   - Serve with lemon wedges.

**Nutrition Info (per serving)**
- Calories: 310
- Protein: 35g
- Carbohydrates: 8g
- Fiber: 1g
- Sugars: 0g
- Total Fat: 15g
- Saturated Fat: 4g
- Cholesterol: 80mg
- Sodium: 220mg

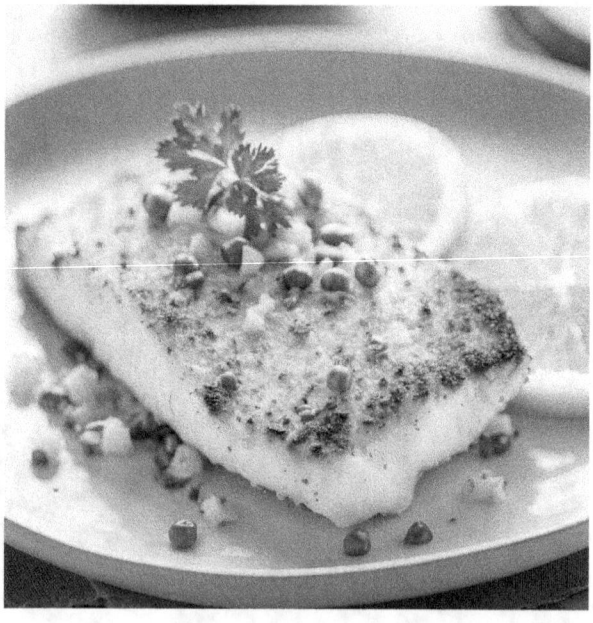

## 21. Spicy Tuna Roll

**Servings:** 4
**Cooking Time:** 30 minutes

**Ingredients**

- 1 cup sushi rice
- 1 1/4 cups water
- 2 tablespoons rice vinegar
- 1 tablespoon sugar
- 1 teaspoon soy sauce
- 1 pound sushi-grade tuna, finely chopped
- 2 tablespoons sriracha
- 1 avocado, sliced
- 4 sheets nori (seaweed)
- 1 cucumber, julienned
- 1 tablespoon sesame seeds
- Soy sauce (for serving)
- Pickled ginger (for serving)

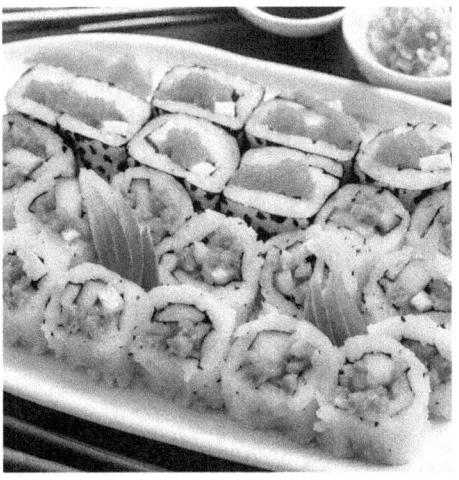

**Instructions**

1. Prepare the Rice:
   - Rinse the sushi rice under cold water until the water runs clear.
   - In a medium saucepan, combine the rice and water. Bring to a boil, then reduce heat to low, cover, and cook for 15 minutes.
   - Remove from heat and let sit, covered, for 10 minutes.
2. Season the Rice:
   - In a small bowl, mix the rice vinegar, sugar, and soy sauce until dissolved.
   - Stir the mixture into the cooked rice and let cool to room temperature.
3. Prepare the Tuna:
   - In a bowl, combine the chopped tuna and sriracha.
4. Assemble the Rolls:
   - Place a sheet of nori on a bamboo sushi mat.
   - Spread a thin layer of rice over the nori, leaving a 1-inch border at the top.
   - Arrange the tuna mixture, avocado slices, and cucumber strips in a line along the bottom edge of the nori.
   - Roll the sushi tightly, using the mat to help.
   - Slice each roll into 6-8 pieces.
5. Serve:
   - Sprinkle sesame seeds over the rolls.
   - Serve with soy sauce and pickled ginger.

**Nutrition Info (per serving)**

- Calories: 320   Protein: 22g   Carbohydrates: 45g   Fiber: 4g
- Sugars: 3g   Total Fat: 8g   Saturated Fat: 1.5g   Cholesterol: 30mg   Sodium: 380mg

## 22. Fish Curry

**Servings:** 4
**Cooking Time:** 30 minutes

**Ingredients**
- 1 pound white fish fillets (such as cod or tilapia), cut into chunks
- 2 tablespoons olive oil
- 1 onion, chopped
- 2 cloves garlic, minced
- 1 tablespoon grated fresh ginger
- 2 tablespoons curry powder
- 1 can (14.5 ounces) diced tomatoes
- 1 can (14 ounces) coconut milk
- 1 cup spinach leaves
- 1 tablespoon lime juice
- Freshly ground black pepper
- Fresh cilantro (optional, for garnish)

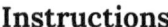

**Instructions**
1. Prepare the Curry Base:
   - In a large skillet, heat the olive oil over medium heat.
   - Add the onion and cook for 3-4 minutes until softened.
   - Add the garlic and ginger, cooking for another 1-2 minutes until fragrant.
   - Stir in the curry powder.
2. Add Liquids and Simmer:
   - Add the diced tomatoes and coconut milk to the skillet.
   - Bring to a simmer and cook for 10 minutes.
3. Cook the Fish:
   - Add the fish chunks to the skillet and simmer for 5-7 minutes until the fish is cooked through and flakes easily.
   - Stir in the spinach leaves and lime juice, cooking until the spinach is wilted.
   - Season with freshly ground black pepper.
4. Serve:
   - Garnish with fresh cilantro if desired.

**Nutrition Info (per serving)**
- Calories: 320
- Protein: 25g
- Carbohydrates: 14g
- Fiber: 3g
- Sugars: 6g
- Total Fat: 18g
- Saturated Fat: 12g
- Cholesterol: 70mg
- Sodium: 180mg

## 23. Grilled Shrimp and Vegetable Bowl

**Servings:** 4
**Cooking Time:** 20 minutes

**Ingredients**
- 1 pound large shrimp, peeled and deveined
- 2 tablespoons olive oil
- 1 teaspoon ground cumin
- 1 teaspoon smoked paprika
- 1 zucchini, sliced
- 1 red bell pepper, sliced
- 1 yellow bell pepper, sliced
- 1 cup cherry tomatoes, halved
- 2 cups cooked quinoa
- 1 avocado, sliced
- Freshly ground black pepper
- Lime wedges (for serving)

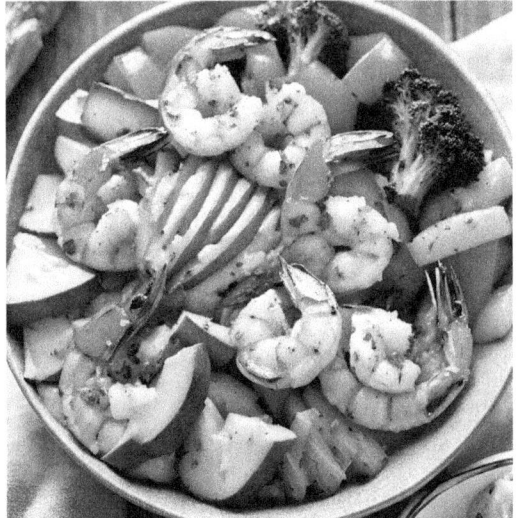

**Instructions**
1. Prepare the Shrimp and Vegetables:
   - Preheat the grill to medium-high heat.
   - Toss the shrimp with 1 tablespoon of olive oil, ground cumin, smoked paprika, and freshly ground black pepper.
   - Toss the zucchini, bell peppers, and cherry tomatoes with the remaining olive oil.
2. Grill the Shrimp and Vegetables:
   - Grill the shrimp for 2-3 minutes on each side until pink and opaque.
   - Grill the vegetables for 5-7 minutes until tender and slightly charred.
3. Assemble the Bowls:
   - Divide the cooked quinoa among four bowls.
   - Top with grilled shrimp, vegetables, and avocado slices.
4. Serve:
   - Serve with lime wedges.

**Nutrition Info (per serving)**
- Calories: 360
- Protein: 28g
- Carbohydrates: 30g
- Fiber: 8g
- Sugars: 6g
- Total Fat: 14g
- Saturated Fat: 2g
- Cholesterol: 190mg
- Sodium: 280mg

## 24. Salmon and Spinach Quiche

**Servings:** 6
**Cooking Time:** 45 minutes

### Ingredients
- 1 pre-made whole wheat pie crust
- 6 ounces cooked salmon, flaked
- 1 cup fresh spinach, chopped
- 1/2 cup grated Swiss cheese
- 4 large eggs
- 1 cup unsweetened almond milk (or any preferred non-dairy milk)
- 1 tablespoon fresh dill, chopped
- Freshly ground black pepper

### Instructions
1. Preheat Oven:
   - Preheat your oven to 375°F (190°C).
2. Prepare the Filling:
   - In a bowl, whisk together the eggs, almond milk, fresh dill, and freshly ground black pepper.
   - Stir in the flaked salmon, chopped spinach, and grated Swiss cheese.
3. Assemble the Quiche:
   - Place the pie crust in a pie dish.
   - Pour the filling into the crust.
4. Bake:
   - Bake for 35-40 minutes, or until the quiche is set and golden brown on top.
5. Serve:
   - Let cool slightly before slicing and serving.

### Nutrition Info (per serving)
- Calories: 300
- Protein: 18g
- Carbohydrates: 20g
- Fiber: 3g
- Sugars: 2g
- Total Fat: 17g
- Saturated Fat: 5g
- Cholesterol: 170mg
- Sodium: 240mg

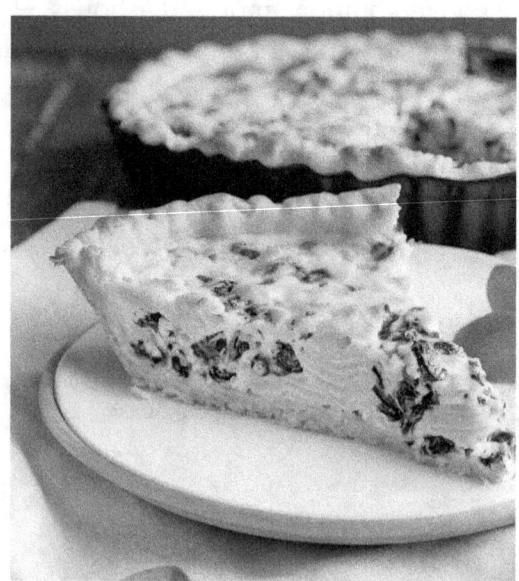

## 25. Kedgeree

**Servings:** 4
**Cooking Time:** 30 minutes

**Ingredients**

- 1 pound smoked haddock fillets
- 1 cup basmati rice
- 4 large eggs
- 1 onion, finely chopped
- 2 tablespoons olive oil
- 1 tablespoon curry powder
- 1/4 cup fresh parsley, chopped
- Freshly ground black pepper
- Lemon wedges (for serving)

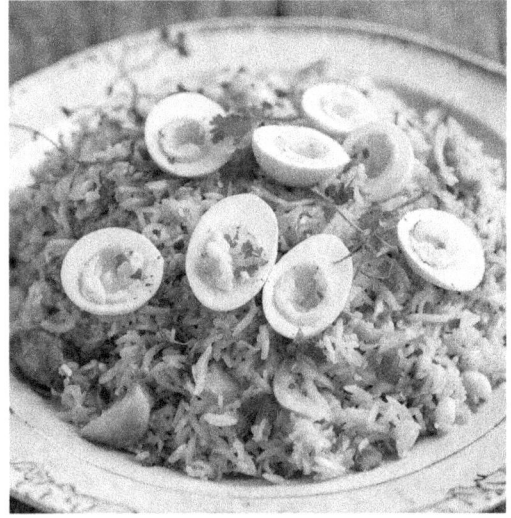

**Instructions**

1. Cook the Rice:
   - Cook the basmati rice according to package instructions.
2. Poach the Haddock:
   - In a large skillet, poach the haddock in simmering water for 10 minutes until cooked through.
   - Remove from water and flake into bite-sized pieces.
3. Boil the Eggs:
   - Boil the eggs for 10 minutes, then peel and quarter them.
4. Prepare the Onion:
   - In a large skillet, heat the olive oil over medium heat.
   - Add the chopped onion and cook for 3-4 minutes until softened.
   - Stir in the curry powder and cook for another minute.
5. Combine and Serve:
   - Add the cooked rice, flaked haddock, and fresh parsley to the skillet. Stir to combine and heat through.
   - Garnish with quartered eggs and freshly ground black pepper.
   - Serve with lemon wedges.

**Nutrition Info (per serving)**

- Calories: 350
- Protein: 27g
- Carbohydrates: 32g
- Fiber: 2g
- Sugars: 3g
- Total Fat: 13g
- Saturated Fat: 3g
- Cholesterol: 220mg
- Sodium: 600mg

## 26. Seafood Fettuccine

**Servings:** 4
**Cooking Time:** 25 minutes

**Ingredients**
- 8 ounces whole wheat fettuccine
- 1 pound mixed seafood (shrimp, scallops, mussels)
- 2 tablespoons olive oil
- 3 cloves garlic, minced
- 1/2 cup dry white wine
- 1 cup low-sodium vegetable broth
- 1/2 cup cherry tomatoes, halved
- 1/4 cup fresh parsley, chopped
- 1/4 cup grated Parmesan cheese
- Freshly ground black pepper
- Lemon wedges (for serving)

**Instructions**
1. Cook the Fettuccine:
   - Cook the fettuccine according to package instructions. Drain and set aside.
2. Cook the Seafood:
   - In a large skillet, heat the olive oil over medium-high heat.
   - Add the minced garlic and cook for 1-2 minutes until fragrant.
   - Add the mixed seafood and cook for 3-4 minutes until the seafood is just cooked through.
3. Prepare the Sauce:
   - Add the white wine and vegetable broth to the skillet. Bring to a simmer and cook for 5 minutes until the sauce is slightly reduced.
   - Stir in the cherry tomatoes and cook for another 2 minutes.
4. Combine and Serve:
   - Add the cooked fettuccine to the skillet and toss to coat with the sauce.
   - Sprinkle with fresh parsley, grated Parmesan cheese, and freshly ground black pepper.
   - Serve with lemon wedges.

**Nutrition Info (per serving)**
- Calories: 380
- Protein: 28g
- Carbohydrates: 45g
- Fiber: 6g
- Sugars: 5g
- Total Fat: 10g
- Saturated Fat: 2g
- Cholesterol: 135mg
- Sodium: 420mg

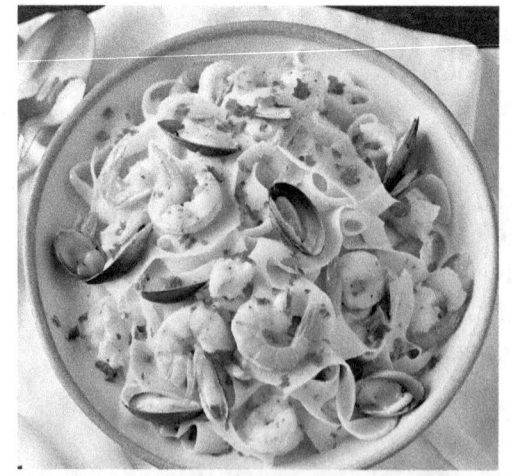

# Vegetables

**1. Roasted Brussels Sprouts with Balsamic Glaze**
**Servings: 4**
**Cooking Time: 30 minutes**
**Ingredients**

- 1 pound Brussels sprouts, trimmed and halved
- 2 tablespoons olive oil
- 1/4 cup balsamic vinegar
- 1 tablespoon honey
- 1/4 cup chopped walnuts
- Freshly ground black pepper

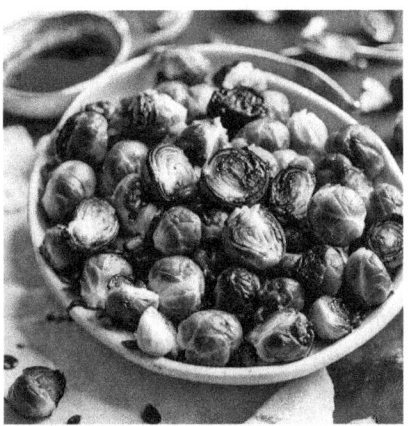

**Instructions**

1. Preheat Oven:
   - Preheat your oven to 400°F (200°C).
2. Prepare the Brussels Sprouts:
   - In a large bowl, toss the Brussels sprouts with olive oil and freshly ground black pepper.
3. Roast the Brussels Sprouts:
   - Spread the Brussels sprouts on a baking sheet in a single layer.
   - Roast for 20-25 minutes, or until tender and caramelized, stirring halfway through.
4. Prepare the Balsamic Glaze:
   - While the Brussels sprouts are roasting, heat the balsamic vinegar and honey in a small saucepan over medium heat.
   - Bring to a simmer and cook for 5-7 minutes until the mixture has reduced and thickened.
5. Combine and Serve:
   - Remove the Brussels sprouts from the oven and transfer to a serving bowl.
   - Drizzle with the balsamic glaze and sprinkle with chopped walnuts.
   - Serve immediately.

**Nutrition Info (per serving)**

- Calories: 180   Protein: 4g   Carbohydrates: 20g   Fiber: 5g
- Sugars: 10g
- Total Fat: 10g
- Saturated Fat: 1g
- Cholesterol: 0mg
- Sodium: 35mg

## 2. Spiced Sweet Potato Soup

**Servings:** 4
**Cooking Time:** 35 minutes

**Ingredients**
- 2 large sweet potatoes, peeled and diced
- 1 onion, chopped
- 3 cloves garlic, minced
- 1 tablespoon olive oil
- 1 teaspoon ground cumin
- 1 teaspoon ground coriander
- 1/2 teaspoon ground cinnamon
- 4 cups low-sodium vegetable broth
- 1 cup coconut milk
- Freshly ground black pepper
- Fresh cilantro (optional, for garnish)

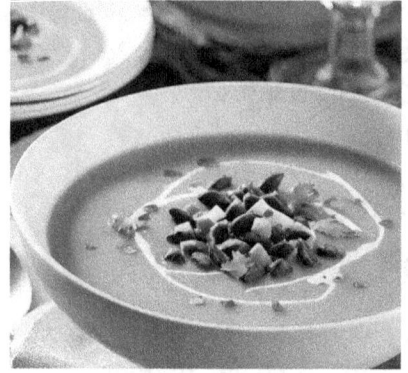

**Instructions**
1. Prepare the Vegetables:
   - In a large pot, heat the olive oil over medium heat.
   - Add the chopped onion and cook for 3-4 minutes until softened.
   - Add the minced garlic and cook for another 1-2 minutes.
2. Add Spices and Sweet Potatoes:
   - Stir in the ground cumin, ground coriander, and ground cinnamon.
   - Add the diced sweet potatoes and stir to coat with the spices.
3. Cook the Soup:
   - Pour in the vegetable broth and bring to a boil.
   - Reduce the heat to low and simmer for 20-25 minutes, or until the sweet potatoes are tender.
4. Blend the Soup:
   - Using an immersion blender, puree the soup until smooth.
   - Stir in the coconut milk and freshly ground black pepper.
5. Serve:
   - Ladle the soup into bowls and garnish with fresh cilantro if desired.

**Nutrition Info (per serving)**
- Calories: 250
- Protein: 3g
- Carbohydrates: 38g
- Fiber: 6g
- Sugars: 9g
- Total Fat: 10g
- Saturated Fat: 6g
- Cholesterol: 0mg
- Sodium: 220mg

## 3. Kale and Quinoa Salad

**Servings: 4**
**Cooking Time: 20 minutes**
**Ingredients**

- 1 cup quinoa
- 2 cups water
- 4 cups chopped kale, stems removed
- 1/2 cup grated carrots
- 1/2 cup diced red bell pepper
- 1/4 cup sunflower seeds
- 1/4 cup dried cranberries
- 3 tablespoons olive oil
- 2 tablespoons lemon juice
- 1 teaspoon Dijon mustard
- 1 teaspoon honey
- Freshly ground black pepper

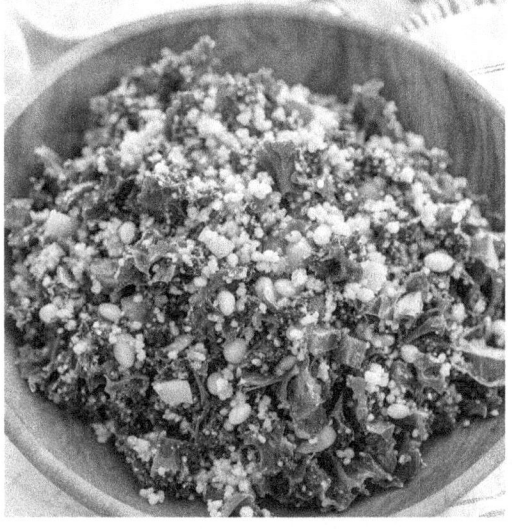

**Instructions**

1. Cook the Quinoa:
    - Rinse the quinoa under cold water.
    - In a medium saucepan, combine the quinoa and water. Bring to a boil, then reduce the heat to low, cover, and simmer for 15 minutes.
    - Remove from heat and let sit, covered, for 5 minutes. Fluff with a fork and let cool.
2. Prepare the Kale:
    - In a large bowl, massage the chopped kale with 1 tablespoon of olive oil until it becomes tender and dark green.
3. Prepare the Dressing:
    - In a small bowl, whisk together the remaining olive oil, lemon juice, Dijon mustard, honey, and freshly ground black pepper.
4. Combine and Serve:
    - In the large bowl with the kale, add the cooled quinoa, grated carrots, diced red bell pepper, sunflower seeds, and dried cranberries.
    - Drizzle with the dressing and toss to combine.
    - Serve immediately.

**Nutrition Info (per serving)**

- Calories: 310   Protein: 8g   Carbohydrates: 38g
- Fiber: 7g
- Sugars: 10g
- Total Fat: 14g
- Saturated Fat: 1.5g
- Cholesterol: 0mg
- Sodium: 45mg

## 4. Grilled Vegetable Platter

**Servings:** 4
**Cooking Time:** 20 minutes

**Ingredients**
- 1 red bell pepper, sliced
- 1 yellow bell pepper, sliced
- 1 zucchini, sliced
- 1 eggplant, sliced
- 1 red onion, sliced
- 2 tablespoons olive oil
- 1 teaspoon dried oregano
- Freshly ground black pepper
- 1 tablespoon balsamic vinegar
- Fresh basil (optional, for garnish)

**Instructions**
1. Prepare the Grill:
   - Preheat the grill to medium-high heat.
2. Prepare the Vegetables:
   - In a large bowl, toss the sliced vegetables with olive oil, dried oregano, and freshly ground black pepper.
3. Grill the Vegetables:
   - Place the vegetables on the grill and cook for 3-4 minutes per side, or until tender and slightly charred.
4. Serve:
   - Arrange the grilled vegetables on a platter.
   - Drizzle with balsamic vinegar and garnish with fresh basil if desired.

**Nutrition Info (per serving)**
- Calories: 150
- Protein: 3g
- Carbohydrates: 18g
- Fiber: 7g
- Sugars: 9g
- Total Fat: 8g
- Saturated Fat: 1g
- Cholesterol: 0mg
- Sodium: 25mg

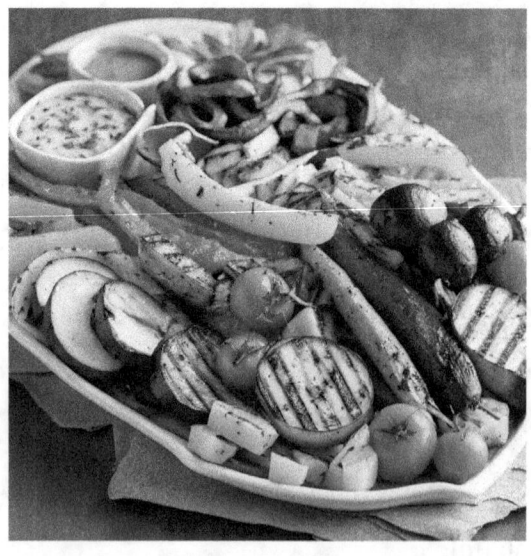

## 5. Carrot and Coriander Soup

**Servings: 4**
**Cooking Time: 30 minutes**
**Ingredients**

- 1 pound carrots, peeled and chopped
- 1 onion, chopped
- 2 cloves garlic, minced
- 1 tablespoon olive oil
- 1 teaspoon ground coriander
- 4 cups low-sodium vegetable broth
- 1/4 cup fresh cilantro, chopped
- Freshly ground black pepper

**Instructions**

1. Prepare the Vegetables:
   - In a large pot, heat the olive oil over medium heat.
   - Add the chopped onion and cook for 3-4 minutes until softened.
   - Add the minced garlic and cook for another 1-2 minutes.
2. Add Spices and Carrots:
   - Stir in the ground coriander.
   - Add the chopped carrots and stir to coat with the spices.
3. Cook the Soup:
   - Pour in the vegetable broth and bring to a boil.
   - Reduce the heat to low and simmer for 20-25 minutes, or until the carrots are tender.
4. Blend the Soup:
   - Using an immersion blender, puree the soup until smooth.
   - Stir in the fresh cilantro and freshly ground black pepper.
5. Serve:
   - Ladle the soup into bowls and garnish with additional cilantro if desired.

**Nutrition Info (per serving)**

- Calories: 160
- Protein: 3g
- Carbohydrates: 26g
- Fiber: 7g
- Sugars: 12g
- Total Fat: 6g
- Saturated Fat: 1g
- Cholesterol: 0mg
- Sodium: 200mg

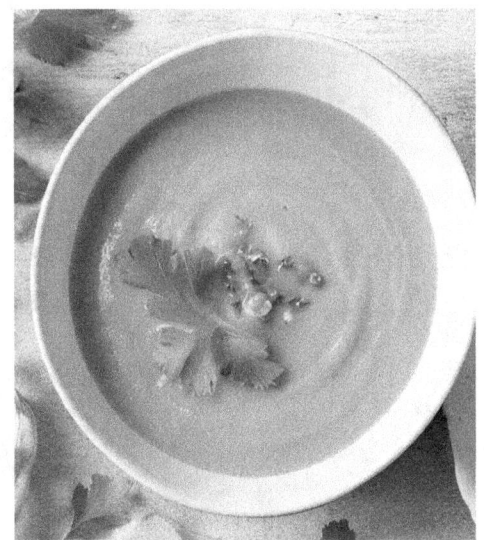

## 6. Zucchini Noodles with Pesto

**Servings:** 4
**Cooking Time:** 20 minutes

**Ingredients**

- 4 large zucchinis, spiralized into noodles
- 2 cups fresh basil leaves
- 1/4 cup pine nuts
- 1/4 cup grated Parmesan cheese
- 2 cloves garlic, minced
- 1/2 cup olive oil
- 1 tablespoon lemon juice
- Freshly ground black pepper
- Cherry tomatoes (optional, for garnish)

**Instructions**

1. Prepare the Pesto:
   - In a food processor, combine the basil leaves, pine nuts, Parmesan cheese, and minced garlic.
   - Pulse until finely chopped.
   - With the processor running, slowly add the olive oil and lemon juice until smooth and well combined.
2. Prepare the Zucchini Noodles:
   - Heat a large skillet over medium heat.
   - Add the zucchini noodles and cook for 3-4 minutes until slightly tender but still crisp.
3. Combine and Serve:
   - Remove the skillet from heat and toss the zucchini noodles with the prepared pesto until evenly coated.
   - Divide among plates and garnish with cherry tomatoes if desired.

**Nutrition Info (per serving)**

- Calories: 240
- Protein: 6g
- Carbohydrates: 8g
- Fiber: 3g
- Sugars: 5g
- Total Fat: 22g
- Saturated Fat: 4g
- Cholesterol: 5mg
- Sodium: 100mg

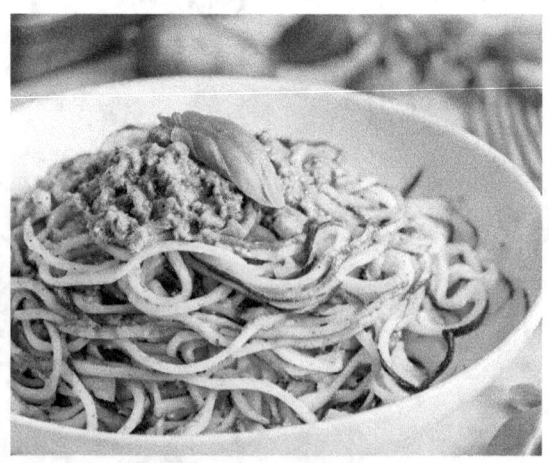

# 7. Cauliflower Steaks with Herb Sauce

**Servings:** 4
**Cooking Time:** 30 minutes

**Ingredients**
- 1 large head of cauliflower, sliced into 1-inch thick steaks
- 3 tablespoons olive oil
- 1 tablespoon lemon juice
- 2 tablespoons chopped fresh parsley
- 1 tablespoon chopped fresh thyme
- 1 tablespoon chopped fresh oregano
- 2 cloves garlic, minced
- Freshly ground black pepper

**Instructions**
1. Preheat Oven:
   - Preheat your oven to 400°F (200°C).
2. Prepare the Cauliflower Steaks:
   - Place the cauliflower steaks on a baking sheet.
   - Brush both sides with 2 tablespoons of olive oil and freshly ground black pepper.
3. Roast the Cauliflower:
   - Roast for 25-30 minutes, flipping halfway through, until the cauliflower is tender and golden brown.
4. Prepare the Herb Sauce:
   - In a small bowl, whisk together the remaining olive oil, lemon juice, parsley, thyme, oregano, and minced garlic.
5. Serve:
   - Drizzle the roasted cauliflower steaks with the herb sauce before serving.

**Nutrition Info (per serving)**
- Calories: 170
- Protein: 4g
- Carbohydrates: 10g
- Fiber: 4g
- Sugars: 4g
- Total Fat: 14g
- Saturated Fat: 2g
- Cholesterol: 0mg
- Sodium: 50mg

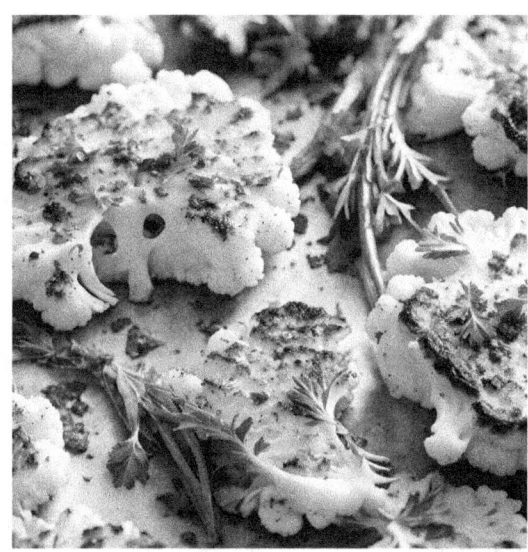

## 8. Eggplant Parmesan

**Servings:** 4
**Cooking Time:** 45 minutes

### Ingredients
- 2 large eggplants, sliced into 1/2-inch rounds
- 1 cup whole wheat bread crumbs
- 1/2 cup grated Parmesan cheese
- 2 eggs, beaten
- 2 cups marinara sauce
- 1 cup shredded mozzarella cheese
- 2 tablespoons olive oil
- Fresh basil (optional, for garnish)

### Instructions
1. Preheat Oven:
   - Preheat your oven to 375°F (190°C).
2. Prepare the Eggplant:
   - In a bowl, mix the bread crumbs and grated Parmesan cheese.
   - Dip each eggplant slice in the beaten eggs, then coat with the bread crumb mixture.
3. Bake the Eggplant:
   - Place the coated eggplant slices on a baking sheet lined with parchment paper.
   - Drizzle with olive oil and bake for 20 minutes, flipping halfway through, until golden brown and tender.
4. Assemble and Bake:
   - Spread a thin layer of marinara sauce in a baking dish.
   - Layer the baked eggplant slices, marinara sauce, and shredded mozzarella cheese.
   - Repeat the layers, finishing with a layer of mozzarella cheese.
   - Bake for 20 minutes, or until the cheese is bubbly and golden.
5. Serve:
   - Garnish with fresh basil if desired.

### Nutrition Info (per serving)
- Calories: 320
- Protein: 15g
- Carbohydrates: 28g
- Fiber: 8g
- Sugars: 10g
- Total Fat: 18g
- Saturated Fat: 6g
- Cholesterol: 75mg
- Sodium: 420mg

## 9. Spaghetti Squash with Tomato Sauce

**Servings:** 4
**Cooking Time:** 40 minutes

**Ingredients**

- 1 large spaghetti squash
- 2 tablespoons olive oil
- 1 onion, chopped
- 3 cloves garlic, minced
- 1 can (14.5 ounces) diced tomatoes
- 1 teaspoon dried oregano
- 1 teaspoon dried basil
- 1/4 teaspoon red pepper flakes (optional)
- Freshly ground black pepper
- Fresh parsley (optional, for garnish)

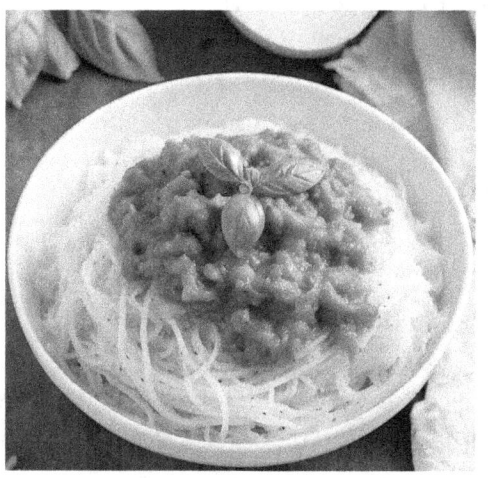

**Instructions**

1. Preheat Oven:
   - Preheat your oven to 375°F (190°C).
2. Prepare the Spaghetti Squash:
   - Cut the spaghetti squash in half lengthwise and remove the seeds.
   - Brush the inside with 1 tablespoon of olive oil and place cut-side down on a baking sheet.
   - Roast for 35-40 minutes, or until the squash is tender.
3. Prepare the Tomato Sauce:
   - In a large skillet, heat the remaining olive oil over medium heat.
   - Add the chopped onion and cook for 3-4 minutes until softened.
   - Add the minced garlic and cook for another 1-2 minutes.
   - Stir in the diced tomatoes, dried oregano, dried basil, red pepper flakes (if using), and freshly ground black pepper.
   - Simmer for 10-15 minutes.
4. Combine and Serve:
   - Using a fork, scrape the roasted spaghetti squash to create strands.
   - Divide the squash among plates and top with the tomato sauce.
   - Garnish with fresh parsley if desired.

**Nutrition Info (per serving)**

- Calories: 180   Protein: 3g
- Carbohydrates: 22g
- Fiber: 6g
- Sugars: 10g
- Total Fat: 9g
- Saturated Fat: 1.5g
- Cholesterol: 0mg
- Sodium: 180mg

## 10. Butternut Squash Risotto

**Servings:** 4
**Cooking Time:** 45 minutes

### Ingredients

- 1 1/2 cups arborio rice
- 4 cups low-sodium vegetable broth
- 1 small onion, finely chopped
- 2 cloves garlic, minced
- 2 tablespoons olive oil
- 1 1/2 cups butternut squash, peeled and diced
- 1/2 cup grated Parmesan cheese
- 1 tablespoon fresh sage, chopped
- Freshly ground black pepper

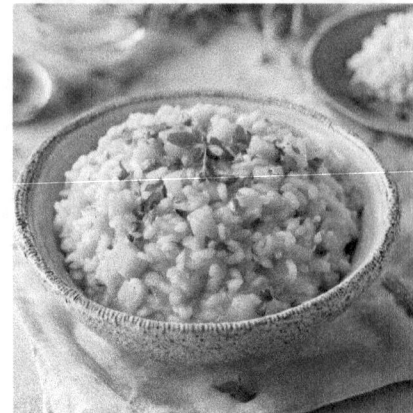

### Instructions

1. Prepare the Broth:
   - In a saucepan, heat the vegetable broth and keep it warm over low heat.
2. Cook the Butternut Squash:
   - In a large skillet, heat 1 tablespoon of olive oil over medium heat.
   - Add the diced butternut squash and cook for 10-12 minutes until tender and slightly caramelized.
   - Remove from the skillet and set aside.
3. Prepare the Risotto:
   - In the same skillet, heat the remaining olive oil over medium heat.
   - Add the chopped onion and cook for 3-4 minutes until softened.
   - Add the minced garlic and cook for another 1-2 minutes.
   - Stir in the arborio rice and cook for 2 minutes until lightly toasted.
4. Add Broth Gradually:
   - Add one ladleful of warm broth to the rice mixture and stir until the liquid is absorbed.
   - Continue adding the broth one ladleful at a time, stirring frequently, until the rice is creamy and tender, about 18-20 minutes.
5. Combine and Serve:
   - Stir in the cooked butternut squash, grated Parmesan cheese, fresh sage, and freshly ground black pepper.
   - Serve immediately.

### Nutrition Info (per serving)

- Calories: 350   Protein: 9g   Carbohydrates: 58g
- Fiber: 5g
- Sugars: 4g
- Total Fat: 10g
- Saturated Fat: 3g
- Cholesterol: 10mg
- Sodium: 260mg

## 11. Curried Lentils with Spinach

**Servings:** 4
**Cooking Time:** 30 minutes

**Ingredients**

- 1 cup dried lentils, rinsed
- 4 cups low-sodium vegetable broth
- 1 onion, finely chopped
- 3 cloves garlic, minced
- 1 tablespoon olive oil
- 1 tablespoon curry powder
- 1 teaspoon ground cumin
- 1 teaspoon ground coriander
- 1 cup canned diced tomatoes
- 4 cups fresh spinach, chopped
- Freshly ground black pepper
- Fresh cilantro (optional, for garnish)

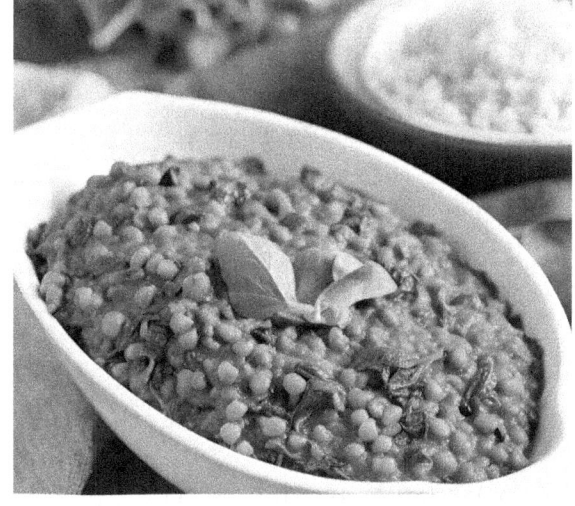

**Instructions**

1. Cook the Lentils:
   - In a large pot, bring the lentils and vegetable broth to a boil.
   - Reduce heat to low, cover, and simmer for 20 minutes, or until the lentils are tender.
2. Prepare the Aromatics:
   - In a large skillet, heat the olive oil over medium heat.
   - Add the chopped onion and cook for 3-4 minutes until softened.
   - Add the minced garlic, curry powder, ground cumin, and ground coriander, cooking for another 1-2 minutes until fragrant.
3. Combine Lentils and Aromatics:
   - Stir the cooked lentils, including their broth, into the skillet with the onions and spices.
   - Add the diced tomatoes and bring to a simmer.
4. Add Spinach and Serve:
   - Stir in the chopped spinach and cook until wilted, about 2-3 minutes.
   - Season with freshly ground black pepper.
   - Garnish with fresh cilantro if desired.

**Nutrition Info (per serving)**

- Calories: 230   Protein: 13g   Carbohydrates: 36g
- Fiber: 14g   Sugars: 7g
- Total Fat: 5g
- Saturated Fat: 0.5g
- Cholesterol: 0mg
- Sodium: 180mg

## 12. Mushroom Stroganoff

**Servings:** 4
**Cooking Time:** 30 minutes

**Ingredients**

- 1 pound mushrooms, sliced
- 1 onion, chopped
- 3 cloves garlic, minced
- 2 tablespoons olive oil
- 1 tablespoon flour
- 1 cup low-sodium vegetable broth
- 1/2 cup unsweetened almond milk (or any preferred non-dairy milk)
- 1 teaspoon Dijon mustard
- 1 teaspoon paprika
- 1/4 cup chopped fresh parsley
- Freshly ground black pepper
- 4 cups cooked whole wheat pasta or rice (for serving)

**Instructions**

1. Cook the Mushrooms and Onions:
   - In a large skillet, heat the olive oil over medium heat.
   - Add the chopped onion and cook for 3-4 minutes until softened.
   - Add the sliced mushrooms and cook for 5-7 minutes until they release their moisture and start to brown.
   - Add the minced garlic and cook for another 1-2 minutes.
2. Prepare the Sauce:
   - Sprinkle the flour over the mushroom mixture and stir to combine.
   - Gradually add the vegetable broth, stirring continuously until the sauce thickens.
   - Stir in the almond milk, Dijon mustard, and paprika.
   - Simmer for 5-7 minutes until the sauce is well combined and thickened.
3. Finish and Serve:
   - Stir in the chopped fresh parsley and freshly ground black pepper.
   - Serve over cooked whole wheat pasta or rice.

**Nutrition Info (per serving)**

- Calories: 280
- Protein: 10g
- Carbohydrates: 40g
- Fiber: 6g
- Sugars: 7g
- Total Fat: 10g
- Saturated Fat: 1.5g
- Cholesterol: 0mg
- Sodium: 200mg

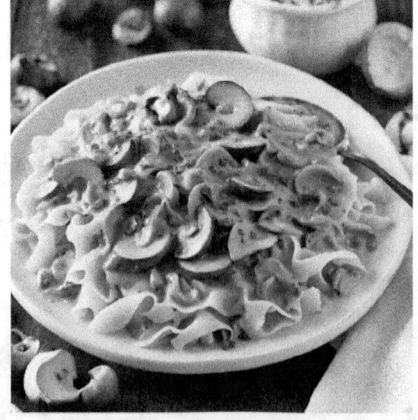

## 13. Garlic Green Beans

**Servings:** 4
**Cooking Time:** 15 minutes

**Ingredients**

- 1 pound green beans, trimmed
- 2 tablespoons olive oil
- 3 cloves garlic, minced
- 1 teaspoon lemon zest
- Freshly ground black pepper
- 1 tablespoon lemon juice
- Fresh parsley (optional, for garnish)

**Instructions**

1. Blanch the Green Beans:
   - Bring a large pot of water to a boil.
   - Add the green beans and cook for 3-4 minutes until tender-crisp.
   - Drain and rinse under cold water to stop the cooking process.
2. Prepare the Garlic Oil:
   - In a large skillet, heat the olive oil over medium heat.
   - Add the minced garlic and cook for 1-2 minutes until fragrant.
3. Combine and Serve:
   - Add the blanched green beans to the skillet and toss to coat with the garlic oil.
   - Stir in the lemon zest and freshly ground black pepper.
   - Cook for another 2-3 minutes until the green beans are heated through.
   - Drizzle with lemon juice and garnish with fresh parsley if desired.

**Nutrition Info (per serving)**

- Calories: 100
- Protein: 2g
- Carbohydrates: 8g
- Fiber: 4g
- Sugars: 3g
- Total Fat: 7g
- Saturated Fat: 1g
- Cholesterol: 0mg
- Sodium: 5mg

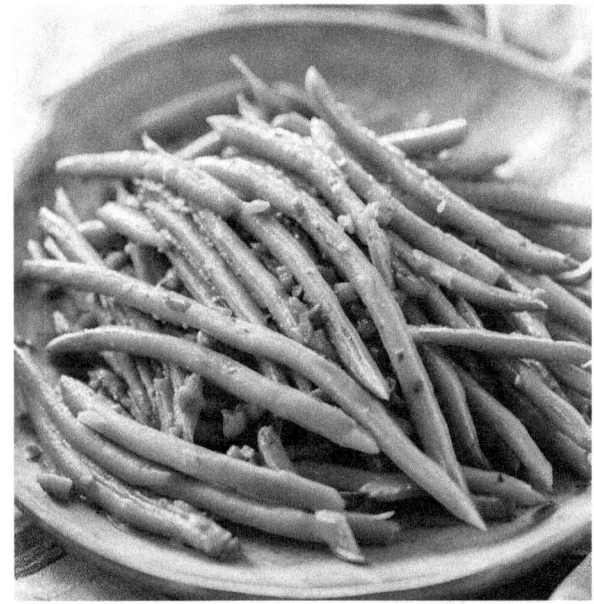

## 14. Vegetable Stir-Fry with Tofu

**Servings:** 4
**Cooking Time:** 20 minutes

### Ingredients

- 1 block (14 ounces) firm tofu, drained and cubed
- 2 tablespoons olive oil
- 1 red bell pepper, sliced
- 1 yellow bell pepper, sliced
- 1 zucchini, sliced
- 1 cup broccoli florets
- 2 cloves garlic, minced
- 1 tablespoon fresh ginger, grated
- 1/4 cup low-sodium soy sauce
- 1 tablespoon rice vinegar
- 1 tablespoon sesame oil
- 1 tablespoon sesame seeds
- Freshly ground black pepper
- 2 cups cooked brown rice (for serving)

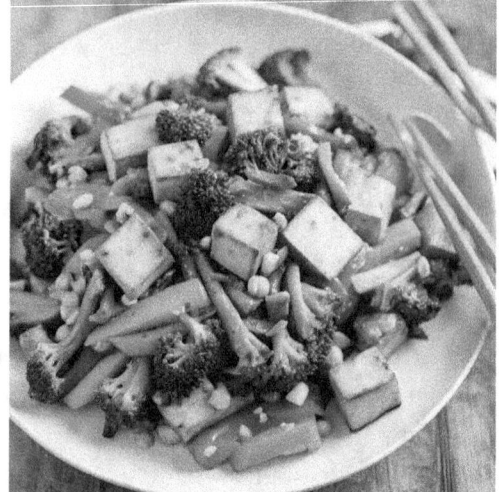

### Instructions

1. Cook the Tofu:
   - In a large skillet or wok, heat 1 tablespoon of olive oil over medium-high heat.
   - Add the cubed tofu and cook for 5-7 minutes until golden brown on all sides.
   - Remove the tofu from the skillet and set aside.
2. Cook the Vegetables:
   - In the same skillet, add the remaining olive oil.
   - Add the bell peppers, zucchini, and broccoli florets.
   - Stir-fry for 5-7 minutes until the vegetables are tender-crisp.
   - Add the minced garlic and grated ginger, cooking for another 1-2 minutes.
3. Combine and Serve:
   - Return the tofu to the skillet.
   - Stir in the soy sauce, rice vinegar, and sesame oil.
   - Cook for another 2-3 minutes until everything is well combined and heated through.
   - Sprinkle with sesame seeds and freshly ground black pepper.
   - Serve over cooked brown rice.

### Nutrition Info (per serving)

- Calories: 300   Protein: 15g   Carbohydrates: 30g   Fiber: 6g
- Sugars: 6g
- Total Fat: 14g
- Saturated Fat: 2g
- Cholesterol: 0mg
- Sodium: 480mg

## 15. Tomato Gazpacho

**Servings:** 4
**Cooking Time:** 15 minutes (plus chilling time)

**Ingredients**
- 6 ripe tomatoes, chopped
- 1 cucumber, peeled and chopped
- 1 red bell pepper, chopped
- 1 small red onion, chopped
- 2 cloves garlic, minced
- 3 tablespoons olive oil
- 2 tablespoons red wine vinegar
- 1 teaspoon ground cumin
- Freshly ground black pepper
- 1 cup low-sodium vegetable broth
- Fresh basil (optional, for garnish)

**Instructions**
1. Blend the Vegetables:
    - In a blender, combine the tomatoes, cucumber, red bell pepper, red onion, and minced garlic.
    - Blend until smooth.
2. Prepare the Gazpacho:
    - Add the olive oil, red wine vinegar, ground cumin, and freshly ground black pepper to the blender.
    - Blend again until well combined.
    - Stir in the vegetable broth.
3. Chill and Serve:
    - Transfer the gazpacho to a large bowl and chill in the refrigerator for at least 2 hours before serving.
    - Garnish with fresh basil if desired.

**Nutrition Info (per serving)**
- Calories: 120
- Protein: 2g
- Carbohydrates: 15g
- Fiber: 4g
- Sugars: 10g
- Total Fat: 8g
- Saturated Fat: 1g
- Cholesterol: 0mg
- Sodium: 120mg

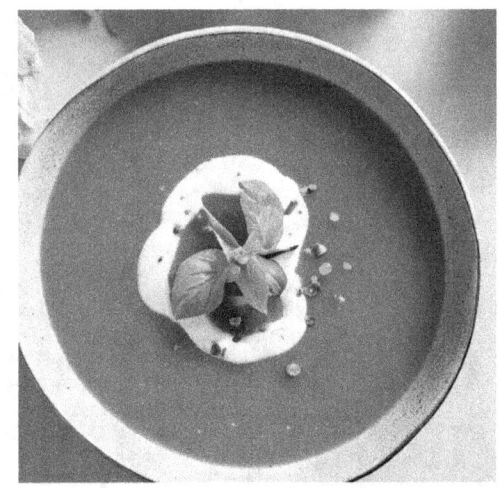

## 16. Cabbage Slaw with Sesame Dressing

**Servings:** 4
**Cooking Time:** 15 minutes

**Ingredients**
- 4 cups shredded cabbage (red and green mix)
- 1 cup shredded carrots
- 1/2 cup sliced green onions
- 1/4 cup chopped fresh cilantro
- 2 tablespoons sesame seeds
- 3 tablespoons rice vinegar
- 2 tablespoons sesame oil
- 1 tablespoon honey
- 1 tablespoon soy sauce
- 1 teaspoon grated fresh ginger
- Freshly ground black pepper

**Instructions**
1. Prepare the Slaw:
   - In a large bowl, combine the shredded cabbage, shredded carrots, sliced green onions, and chopped cilantro.
2. Prepare the Dressing:
   - In a small bowl, whisk together the rice vinegar, sesame oil, honey, soy sauce, grated ginger, and freshly ground black pepper.
3. Combine and Serve:
   - Pour the dressing over the slaw mixture and toss to combine.
   - Sprinkle with sesame seeds before serving.

**Nutrition Info (per serving)**
- Calories: 120
- Protein: 2g
- Carbohydrates: 12g
- Fiber: 4g
- Sugars: 7g
- Total Fat: 7g
- Saturated Fat: 1g
- Cholesterol: 0mg
- Sodium: 180mg

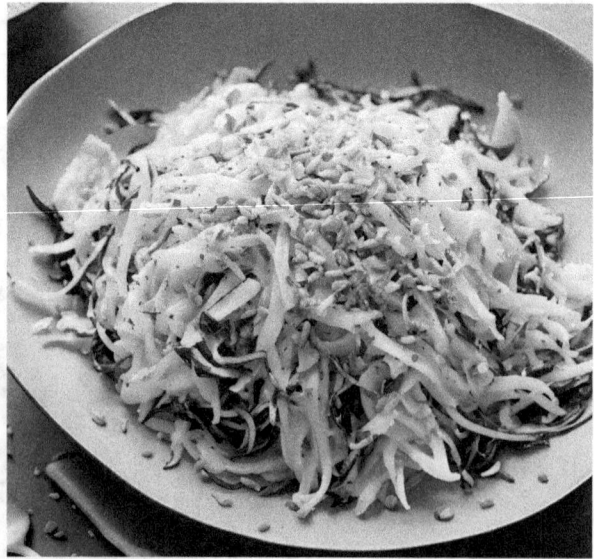

## 17. Roasted Turnips with Rosemary

**Servings:** 4
**Cooking Time:** 30 minutes

**Ingredients**
- 1 1/2 pounds turnips, peeled and diced
- 2 tablespoons olive oil
- 1 teaspoon dried rosemary
- Freshly ground black pepper
- 1 tablespoon lemon juice
- Fresh parsley (optional, for garnish)

**Instructions**
1. Preheat Oven:
   - Preheat your oven to 400°F (200°C).
2. Prepare the Turnips:
   - In a large bowl, toss the diced turnips with olive oil, dried rosemary, and freshly ground black pepper.
3. Roast the Turnips:
   - Spread the turnips on a baking sheet in a single layer.
   - Roast for 25-30 minutes, or until tender and golden brown, stirring halfway through.
4. Serve:
   - Drizzle with lemon juice and garnish with fresh parsley if desired.

**Nutrition Info (per serving)**
- Calories: 110
- Protein: 2g
- Carbohydrates: 14g
- Fiber: 4g
- Sugars: 7g
- Total Fat: 6g
- Saturated Fat: 1g
- Cholesterol: 0mg
- Sodium: 35mg

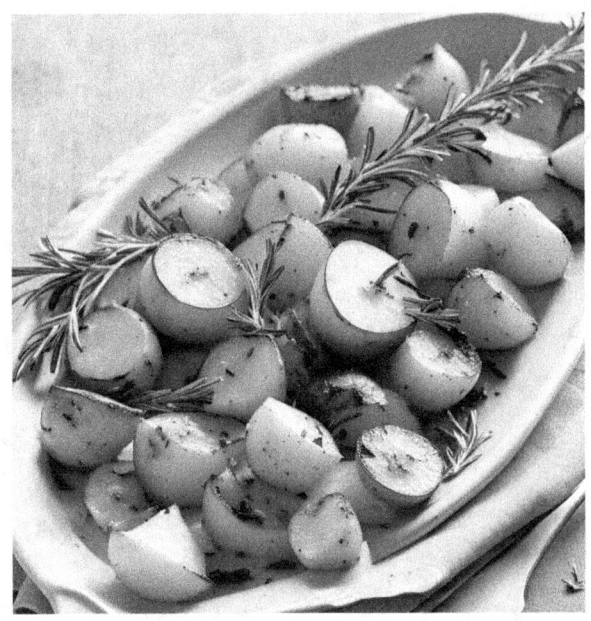

## 18. Sautéed Swiss Chard with Pine Nuts

**Servings:** 4
**Cooking Time:** 15 minutes

**Ingredients**
- 1 bunch Swiss chard, stems removed and leaves chopped
- 3 cloves garlic, minced
- 2 tablespoons olive oil
- 1/4 cup pine nuts
- 1 tablespoon lemon juice
- Freshly ground black pepper

**Instructions**
1. Toast the Pine Nuts:
   - In a dry skillet, toast the pine nuts over medium heat until golden brown, about 2-3 minutes. Remove and set aside.
2. Sauté the Swiss Chard:
   - In the same skillet, heat the olive oil over medium heat.
   - Add the minced garlic and cook for 1-2 minutes until fragrant.
   - Add the chopped Swiss chard and cook for 5-7 minutes until wilted and tender.
3. Combine and Serve:
   - Stir in the toasted pine nuts and lemon juice.
   - Season with freshly ground black pepper before serving.

**Nutrition Info (per serving)**
- Calories: 140
- Protein: 3g
- Carbohydrates: 8g
- Fiber: 4g
- Sugars: 2g
- Total Fat: 11g
- Saturated Fat: 1.5g
- Cholesterol: 0mg
- Sodium: 60mg

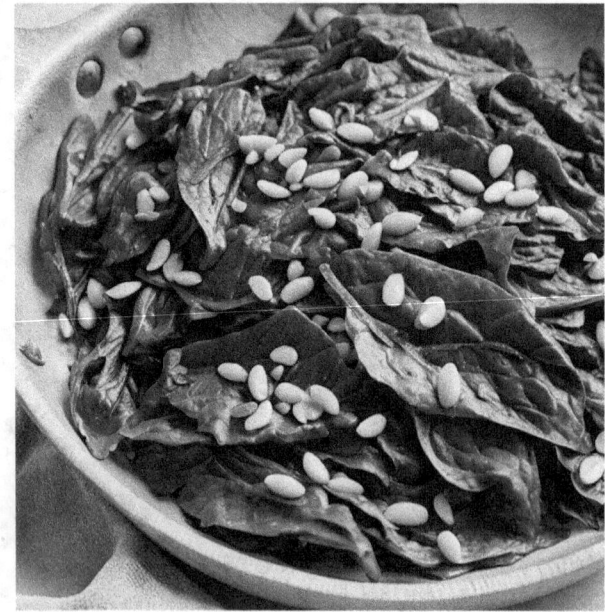

## 19. Vegan Ratatouille

**Servings:** 4
**Cooking Time:** 45 minutes

**Ingredients**

- 1 eggplant, diced
- 1 zucchini, diced
- 1 yellow squash, diced
- 1 red bell pepper, diced
- 1 onion, chopped
- 3 cloves garlic, minced
- 2 tablespoons olive oil
- 1 can (14.5 ounces) diced tomatoes
- 1 teaspoon dried thyme
- 1 teaspoon dried basil
- 1/2 teaspoon dried oregano
- Freshly ground black pepper
- Fresh basil (optional, for garnish)

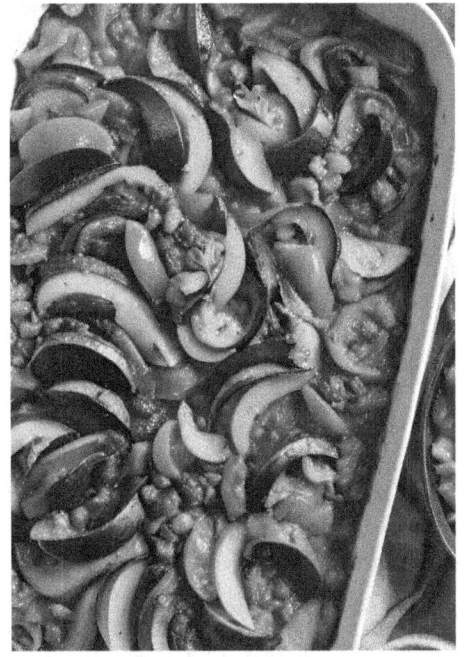

**Instructions**

1. Preheat Oven:
   - Preheat your oven to 375°F (190°C).
2. Prepare the Vegetables:
   - In a large ovenproof skillet or baking dish, combine the diced eggplant, zucchini, yellow squash, red bell pepper, and chopped onion.
   - Toss with olive oil, minced garlic, dried thyme, dried basil, dried oregano, and freshly ground black pepper.
3. Bake the Ratatouille:
   - Pour the diced tomatoes over the vegetable mixture and stir to combine.
   - Cover with foil and bake for 30 minutes.
   - Remove the foil and bake for an additional 15 minutes, or until the vegetables are tender and the flavors are well combined.
4. Serve:
   - Garnish with fresh basil if desired.

**Nutrition Info (per serving)**

- Calories: 170   Protein: 3g   Carbohydrates: 22   Fiber: 8g
- Sugars: 12g   Total Fat: 8g   Saturated Fat: 1g
- Cholesterol: 0mg
- Sodium: 200mg

## 20. Spinach and Feta Pie
**Servings:** 6
**Cooking Time:** 45 minutes

### Ingredients
- 1 pre-made whole wheat pie crust
- 1 tablespoon olive oil
- 1 onion, chopped
- 3 cloves garlic, minced
- 6 cups fresh spinach, chopped
- 1/2 cup crumbled feta cheese
- 3 large eggs
- 1 cup unsweetened almond milk (or any preferred non-dairy milk)
- 1 tablespoon fresh dill, chopped
- Freshly ground black pepper

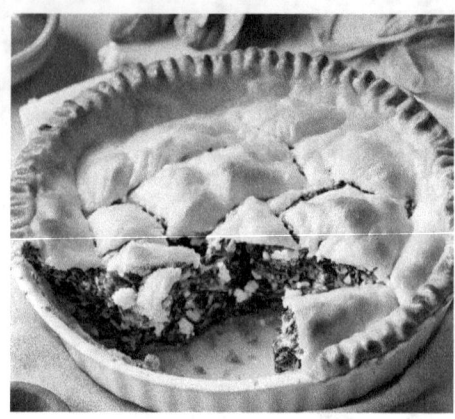

### Instructions
1. Preheat Oven:
    - Preheat your oven to 375°F (190°C).
2. Prepare the Spinach Filling:
    - In a large skillet, heat the olive oil over medium heat.
    - Add the chopped onion and cook for 3-4 minutes until softened.
    - Add the minced garlic and cook for another 1-2 minutes.
    - Stir in the chopped spinach and cook until wilted, about 3-5 minutes.
    - Remove from heat and let cool slightly.
3. Assemble the Pie:
    - In a bowl, whisk together the eggs, almond milk, fresh dill, and freshly ground black pepper.
    - Stir in the cooled spinach mixture and crumbled feta cheese.
    - Pour the filling into the pre-made pie crust.
4. Bake:
    - Bake for 35-40 minutes, or until the pie is set and golden brown on top.
5. Serve:
    - Let the pie cool slightly before slicing and serving.

### Nutrition Info (per serving)
- Calories: 250
- Protein: 9g
- Carbohydrates: 18g
- Fiber: 3g
- Sugars: 2g
- Total Fat: 16g
- Saturated Fat: 5g
- Cholesterol: 110mg
- Sodium: 270mg

## 21. Pumpkin Chili

**Servings:** 4
**Cooking Time:** 40 minutes

**Ingredients**

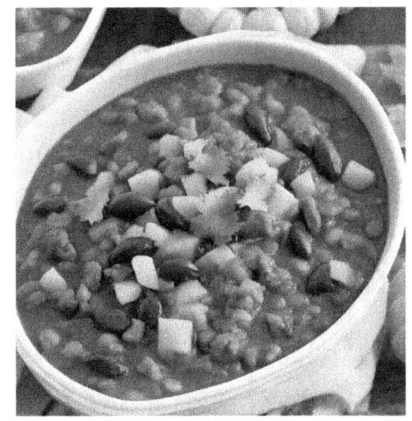

- 1 tablespoon olive oil
- 1 onion, chopped
- 3 cloves garlic, minced
- 1 bell pepper, chopped
- 1 zucchini, chopped
- 1 can (15 ounces) pumpkin puree
- 1 can (15 ounces) black beans, drained and rinsed
- 1 can (15 ounces) kidney beans, drained and rinsed
- 1 can (14.5 ounces) diced tomatoes
- 2 cups low-sodium vegetable broth
- 1 tablespoon chili powder
- 1 teaspoon ground cumin
- 1 teaspoon ground coriander
- Freshly ground black pepper
- Fresh cilantro (optional, for garnish)

**Instructions**

1. Prepare the Aromatics:
   - In a large pot, heat the olive oil over medium heat.
   - Add the chopped onion and cook for 3-4 minutes until softened.
   - Add the minced garlic and cook for another 1-2 minutes.
2. Add Vegetables and Spices:
   - Stir in the chopped bell pepper and zucchini, cooking for another 5 minutes.
   - Add the chili powder, ground cumin, ground coriander, and freshly ground black pepper, stirring to combine.
3. Combine Ingredients:
   - Add the pumpkin puree, black beans, kidney beans, diced tomatoes, and vegetable broth.
   - Bring to a boil, then reduce heat to low and simmer for 25-30 minutes.
4. Serve:
   - Ladle the chili into bowls and garnish with fresh cilantro if desired.

**Nutrition Info (per serving)**

- Calories: 280   Protein: 10g   Carbohydrates: 50g   Fiber: 14g
- Sugars: 10g   Total Fat: 5g
- Saturated Fat: 1g
- Cholesterol: 0mg
- Sodium: 240mg

## 22. Grilled Asparagus with Lemon Tarragon Dressing

**Servings:** 4
**Cooking Time:** 15 minutes

### Ingredients
- 1 pound asparagus, trimmed
- 2 tablespoons olive oil
- 2 tablespoons lemon juice
- 1 teaspoon lemon zest
- 1 teaspoon Dijon mustard
- 1 tablespoon chopped fresh tarragon
- Freshly ground black pepper

### Instructions
1. Prepare the Asparagus:
   - Preheat the grill to medium-high heat.
   - Toss the asparagus with 1 tablespoon of olive oil and freshly ground black pepper.
2. Grill the Asparagus:
   - Grill the asparagus for 3-4 minutes on each side until tender and slightly charred.
3. Prepare the Dressing:
   - In a small bowl, whisk together the lemon juice, lemon zest, Dijon mustard, chopped tarragon, and remaining olive oil.
4. Serve:
   - Drizzle the lemon tarragon dressing over the grilled asparagus before serving.

### Nutrition Info (per serving)
- Calories: 100
- Protein: 2g
- Carbohydrates: 6g
- Fiber: 3g
- Sugars: 2g
- Total Fat: 9g
- Saturated Fat: 1.5g
- Cholesterol: 0mg
- Sodium: 50mg

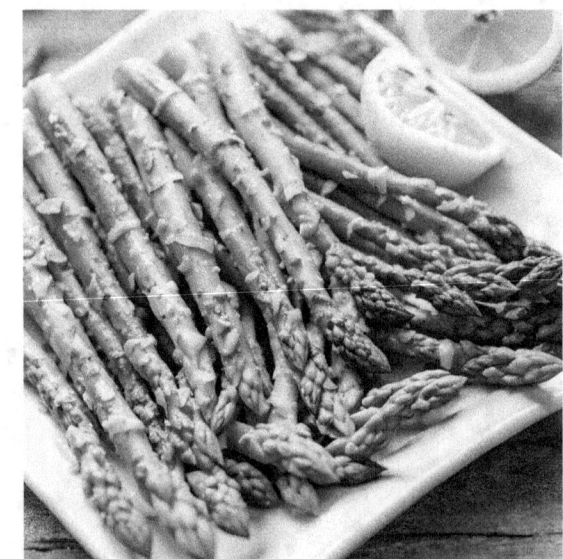

## 23. Vegetable Paella

**Servings:** 4
**Cooking Time:** 45 minutes

**Ingredients**

- 2 tablespoons olive oil
- 1 onion, chopped
- 3 cloves garlic, minced
- 1 red bell pepper, chopped
- 1 yellow bell pepper, chopped
- 1 cup Arborio rice
- 1 can (14.5 ounces) diced tomatoes
- 3 cups low-sodium vegetable broth
- 1 teaspoon smoked paprika
- 1/2 teaspoon turmeric
- 1 cup green beans, trimmed and cut into 1-inch pieces
- 1 cup frozen peas, thawed
- 1/4 cup chopped fresh parsley
- Freshly ground black pepper
- Lemon wedges (for serving)

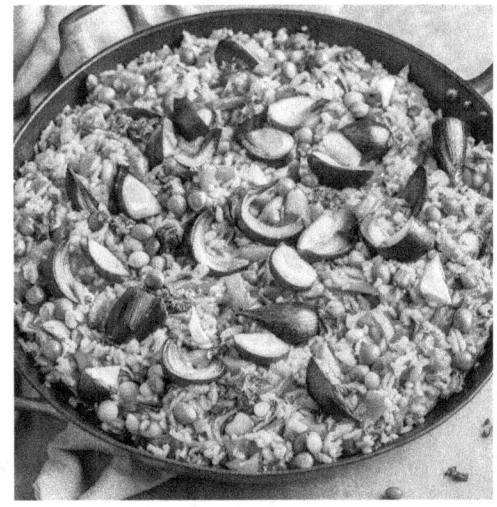

**Instructions**

1. Prepare the Vegetables:
   - In a large skillet or paella pan, heat the olive oil over medium heat.
   - Add the chopped onion and cook for 3-4 minutes until softened.
   - Add the minced garlic, red bell pepper, and yellow bell pepper, cooking for another 5 minutes.
2. Cook the Rice:
   - Stir in the Arborio rice, smoked paprika, turmeric, and freshly ground black pepper.
   - Add the diced tomatoes and vegetable broth, stirring to combine.
   - Bring to a boil, then reduce heat to low and simmer for 20 minutes.
3. Add the Vegetables:
   - Stir in the green beans and peas.
   - Cover and cook for another 10-15 minutes until the rice is tender and the liquid is absorbed.
4. Serve:
   - Garnish with chopped fresh parsley and serve with lemon wedges.

**Nutrition Info (per serving)**

- Calories: 310   Protein: 8g   Carbohydrates: 53g   Fiber: 8g
- Sugars: 8g   Total Fat: 9g   Saturated Fat: 1.5g
- Cholesterol: 0mg
- Sodium: 240mg

## 24. Mashed Cauliflower with Chives

**Servings:** 4
**Cooking Time:** 20 minutes

**Ingredients**
- 1 large head cauliflower, cut into florets
- 2 tablespoons olive oil
- 1/4 cup unsweetened almond milk (or any preferred non-dairy milk)
- 1/4 cup chopped fresh chives
- Freshly ground black pepper

**Instructions**
1. Cook the Cauliflower:
   - Bring a large pot of water to a boil.
   - Add the cauliflower florets and cook for 10-12 minutes until tender.
   - Drain and return to the pot.
2. Mash the Cauliflower:
   - Add the olive oil and almond milk to the cauliflower.
   - Using an immersion blender or potato masher, mash until smooth and creamy.
   - Stir in the chopped chives and freshly ground black pepper.
3. Serve:
   - Transfer to a serving bowl and serve immediately.

**Nutrition Info (per serving)**
- Calories: 100
- Protein: 3g
- Carbohydrates: 10g
- Fiber: 4g
- Sugars: 3g
- Total Fat: 7g
- Saturated Fat: 1g
- Cholesterol: 0mg
- Sodium: 30mg

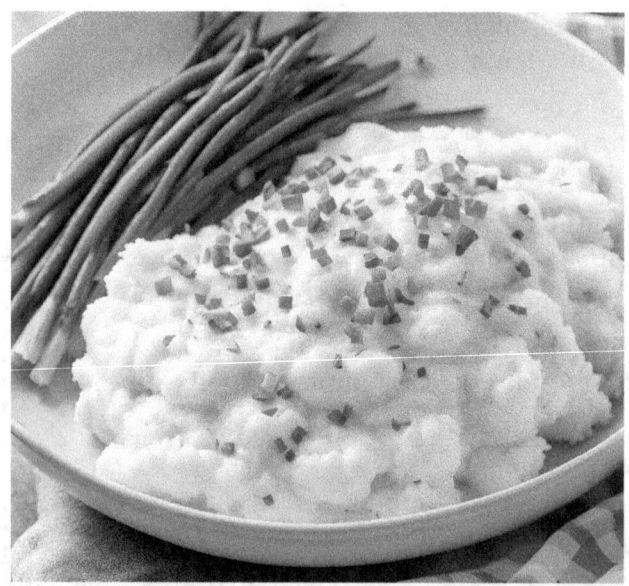

## 25. Roasted Radishes with Soy Sauce

**Servings:** 4
**Cooking Time:** 20 minutes

**Ingredients**

- 1 pound radishes, trimmed and halved
- 2 tablespoons olive oil
- 1 tablespoon soy sauce
- 1 teaspoon ground ginger
- Freshly ground black pepper
- 1 tablespoon sesame seeds
- Fresh cilantro (optional, for garnish)

**Instructions**

1. Preheat Oven:
   - Preheat your oven to 425°F (220°C).
2. Prepare the Radishes:
   - In a large bowl, toss the halved radishes with olive oil, soy sauce, ground ginger, and freshly ground black pepper.
3. Roast the Radishes:
   - Spread the radishes on a baking sheet in a single layer.
   - Roast for 15-20 minutes, or until tender and slightly caramelized.
4. Serve:
   - Sprinkle with sesame seeds and garnish with fresh cilantro if desired.

**Nutrition Info (per serving)**

- Calories: 90
- Protein: 2g
- Carbohydrates: 6g
- Fiber: 3g
- Sugars: 3g
- Total Fat: 7g
- Saturated Fat: 1g
- Cholesterol: 0mg
- Sodium: 150mg

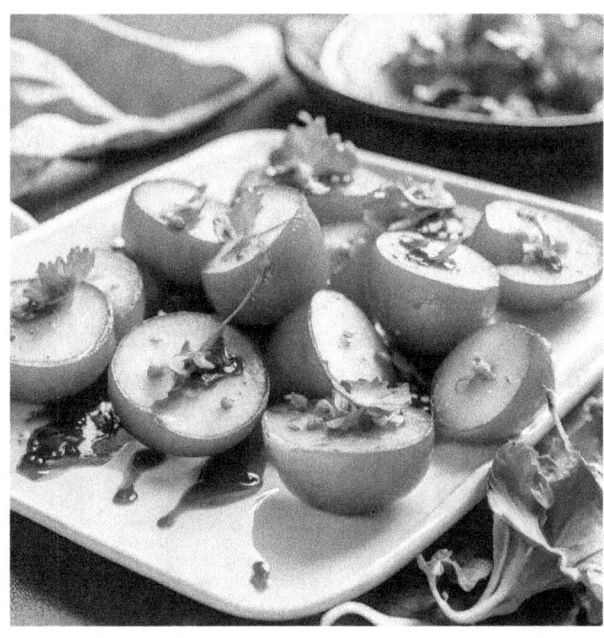

# Poultry Recipes

**1. Grilled Chicken with Avocado Salsa**
**Servings: 4**
**Cooking Time: 25 minutes**
**Ingredients**
- 4 boneless, skinless chicken breasts
- 2 tablespoons olive oil
- 1 teaspoon ground cumin
- 1 teaspoon paprika
- Freshly ground black pepper
- 2 ripe avocados, diced
- 1 cup cherry tomatoes, halved
- 1/4 cup red onion, finely chopped
- 1 tablespoon lime juice
- 2 tablespoons chopped fresh cilantro

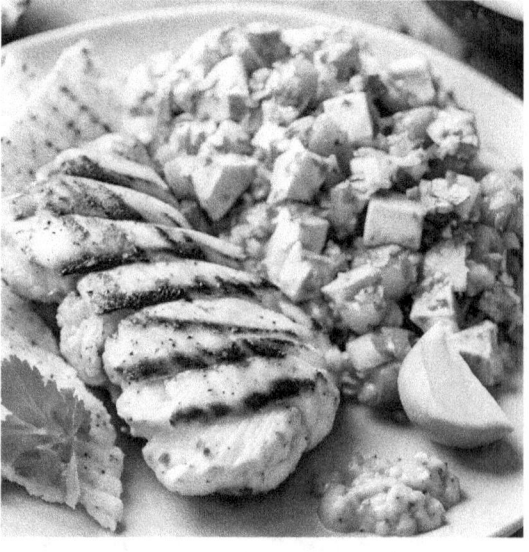

**Instructions**
1. Prepare the Chicken:
   - Preheat the grill to medium-high heat.
   - Brush the chicken breasts with olive oil and sprinkle with ground cumin, paprika, and freshly ground black pepper.
2. Grill the Chicken:
   - Grill the chicken breasts for 6-7 minutes on each side, or until cooked through and the internal temperature reaches 165°F (75°C).
3. Prepare the Avocado Salsa:
   - In a bowl, combine the diced avocados, cherry tomatoes, red onion, lime juice, and chopped cilantro. Mix gently.
4. Serve:
   - Place the grilled chicken on plates and top with the avocado salsa.

**Nutrition Info (per serving)**
- Calories: 350
- Protein: 30g
- Carbohydrates: 12g
- Fiber: 6g
- Sugars: 3g
- Total Fat: 20g
- Saturated Fat: 3g
- Cholesterol: 70mg
- Sodium: 80mg

## 2. Turkey and Spinach Meatballs

**Servings:** 4
**Cooking Time:** 30 minutes
**Ingredients**

- 1 pound ground turkey
- 1 cup fresh spinach, finely chopped
- 1/2 cup whole wheat bread crumbs
- 1/4 cup grated Parmesan cheese
- 1 egg, beaten
- 2 cloves garlic, minced
- 1 teaspoon dried oregano
- Freshly ground black pepper
- 1 tablespoon olive oil

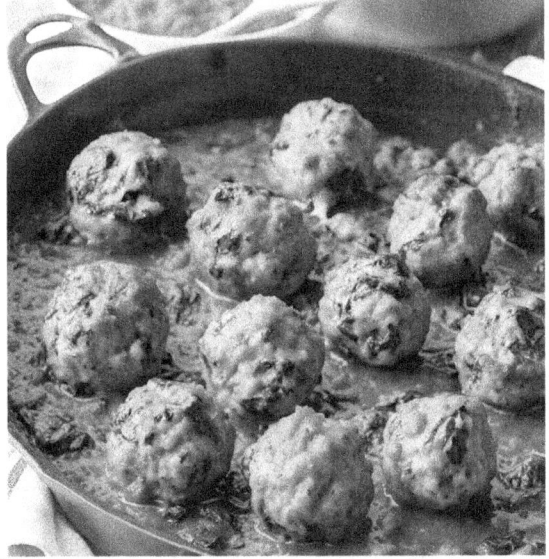

**Instructions**

1. Prepare the Meatballs:
   - Preheat the oven to 375°F (190°C).
   - In a large bowl, combine the ground turkey, chopped spinach, bread crumbs, Parmesan cheese, beaten egg, minced garlic, dried oregano, and freshly ground black pepper. Mix until well combined.
   - Form the mixture into 16 meatballs.
2. Cook the Meatballs:
   - In a large skillet, heat the olive oil over medium-high heat.
   - Add the meatballs and cook for 5-7 minutes, turning occasionally, until browned on all sides.
   - Transfer the meatballs to a baking sheet and bake for 15-20 minutes, or until cooked through and the internal temperature reaches 165°F (75°C).
3. Serve:
   - Serve the meatballs with your favorite sauce or as part of a meal.

**Nutrition Info (per serving)**

- Calories: 280
- Protein: 25g
- Carbohydrates: 10g
- Fiber: 2g
- Sugars: 1g
- Total Fat: 15g
- Saturated Fat: 4g
- Cholesterol: 110mg
- Sodium: 200mg

## 3. Lemon Herb Roasted Chicken

**Servings:** 4
**Cooking Time:** 1 hour 15 minutes

**Ingredients**
- 1 whole chicken (about 4 pounds)
- 1/4 cup olive oil
- 1/4 cup lemon juice
- 2 tablespoons chopped fresh rosemary
- 2 tablespoons chopped fresh thyme
- 4 cloves garlic, minced
- Freshly ground black pepper
- Lemon wedges (for serving)

**Instructions**
1. Prepare the Chicken:
   - Preheat the oven to 375°F (190°C).
   - In a bowl, mix together the olive oil, lemon juice, chopped rosemary, chopped thyme, minced garlic, and freshly ground black pepper.
2. Roast the Chicken:
   - Place the chicken in a roasting pan and rub the lemon herb mixture all over the chicken, including under the skin.
   - Roast in the preheated oven for 1 hour and 15 minutes, or until the internal temperature of the chicken reaches 165°F (75°C).
3. Serve:
   - Let the chicken rest for 10 minutes before carving.
   - Serve with lemon wedges.

**Nutrition Info (per serving)**
- Calories: 450
- Protein: 35g
- Carbohydrates: 2g
- Fiber: 1g
- Sugars: 0g
- Total Fat: 32g
- Saturated Fat: 8g
- Cholesterol: 140mg
- Sodium: 90mg

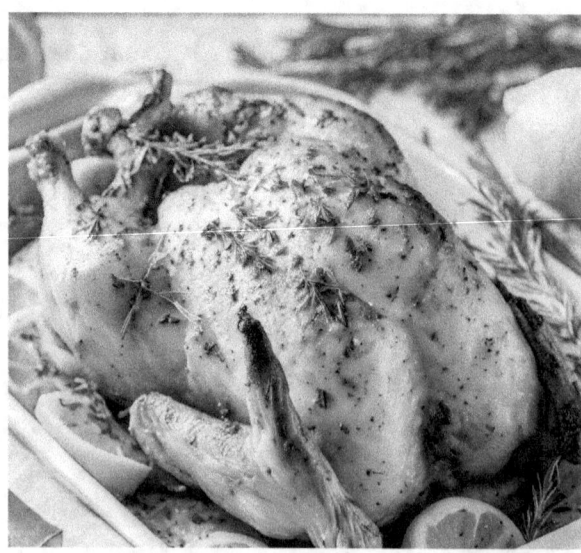

## 4. Chicken Stir-Fry with Broccoli

**Servings:** 4
**Cooking Time:** 25 minutes

**Ingredients**
- 1 pound boneless, skinless chicken breasts, thinly sliced
- 3 tablespoons olive oil
- 2 cloves garlic, minced
- 1 tablespoon fresh ginger, grated
- 4 cups broccoli florets
- 1 red bell pepper, sliced
- 1/4 cup low-sodium soy sauce
- 1 tablespoon rice vinegar
- 1 tablespoon honey
- Freshly ground black pepper

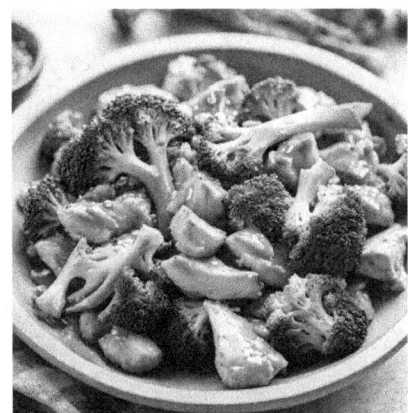

**Instructions**
1. Prepare the Chicken:
   - In a large skillet or wok, heat 2 tablespoons of olive oil over medium-high heat.
   - Add the sliced chicken and cook for 5-7 minutes until browned and cooked through.
   - Remove the chicken from the skillet and set aside.
2. Cook the Vegetables:
   - In the same skillet, add the remaining olive oil.
   - Add the minced garlic and grated ginger, cooking for 1-2 minutes until fragrant.
   - Add the broccoli florets and red bell pepper, cooking for 5-7 minutes until tender-crisp.
3. Combine and Serve:
   - Return the chicken to the skillet.
   - In a small bowl, mix together the soy sauce, rice vinegar, honey, and freshly ground black pepper.
   - Pour the sauce over the chicken and vegetables, tossing to combine and cook for another 2-3 minutes.
   - Serve immediately.

**Nutrition Info (per serving)**
- Calories: 280   Protein: 30g   Carbohydrates: 14g
- Fiber: 4g
- Sugars: 8g
- Total Fat: 12g
- Saturated Fat: 2g
- Cholesterol: 70mg
- Sodium: 450mg

## 5. Baked Pesto Chicken

**Servings:** 4
**Cooking Time:** 30 minutes

**Ingredients**

- 4 boneless, skinless chicken breasts
- 1/2 cup basil pesto
- 1/2 cup cherry tomatoes, halved
- 1/4 cup grated Parmesan cheese
- 2 tablespoons olive oil
- Freshly ground black pepper

**Instructions**

1. Prepare the Chicken:
   - Preheat the oven to 375°F (190°C).
   - Place the chicken breasts in a baking dish and brush with olive oil.
   - Spread the basil pesto evenly over each chicken breast.
   - Top with halved cherry tomatoes and grated Parmesan cheese.
2. Bake the Chicken:
   - Bake in the preheated oven for 25-30 minutes, or until the chicken is cooked through and the internal temperature reaches 165°F (75°C).
3. Serve:
   - Remove from the oven and let rest for 5 minutes before serving.

**Nutrition Info (per serving)**

- Calories: 340
- Protein: 32g
- Carbohydrates: 4g
- Fiber: 1g
- Sugars: 1g
- Total Fat: 20g
- Saturated Fat: 5g
- Cholesterol: 85mg
- Sodium: 260mg

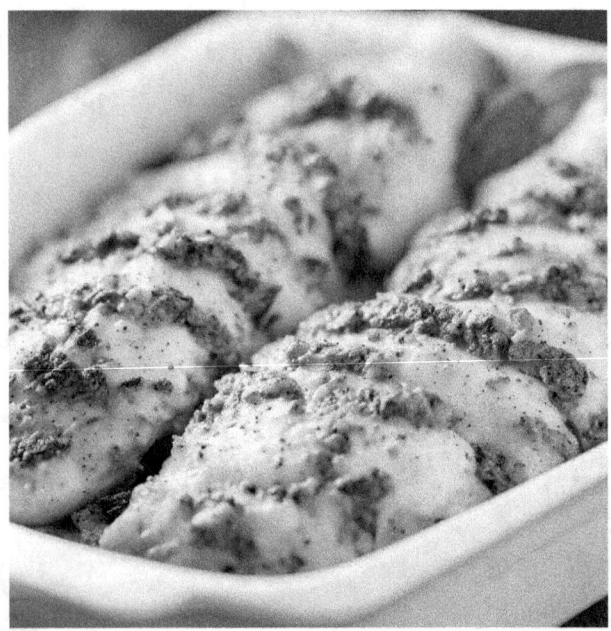

## 6. Smoked Paprika Chicken

**Servings:** 4
**Cooking Time:** 25 minutes

**Ingredients**

- 4 boneless, skinless chicken breasts
- 2 tablespoons olive oil
- 2 teaspoons smoked paprika
- 1 teaspoon garlic powder
- Freshly ground black pepper
- 1 lemon, cut into wedges (for serving)
- Fresh parsley (optional, for garnish)

**Instructions**

1. Prepare the Chicken:
   - Preheat the oven to 375°F (190°C).
   - In a small bowl, mix the smoked paprika, garlic powder, and freshly ground black pepper.
   - Rub the olive oil and spice mixture all over the chicken breasts.
2. Bake the Chicken:
   - Place the chicken breasts on a baking sheet.
   - Bake for 20-25 minutes, or until the chicken is cooked through and the internal temperature reaches 165°F (75°C).
3. Serve:
   - Garnish with lemon wedges and fresh parsley if desired.

**Nutrition Info (per serving)**

- Calories: 270
- Protein: 31g
- Carbohydrates: 2g
- Fiber: 0g
- Sugars: 0g
- Total Fat: 15g
- Saturated Fat: 2.5g
- Cholesterol: 85mg
- Sodium: 90mg

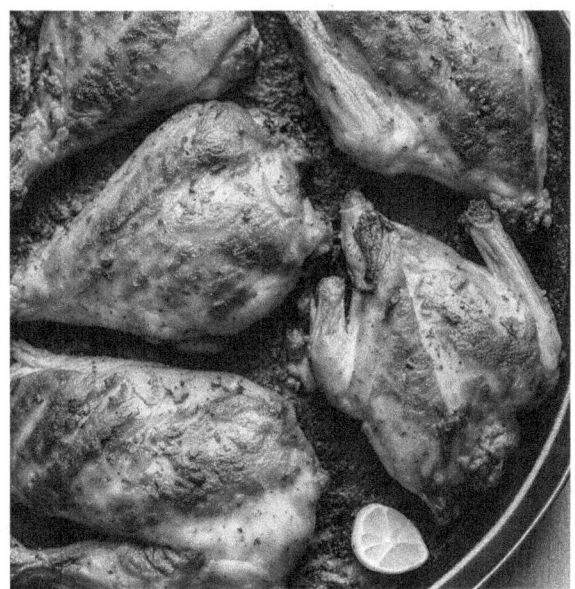

## 7. Asian Turkey Lettuce Wraps

**Servings:** 4
**Cooking Time:** 20 minutes

**Ingredients**

- 1 pound ground turkey
- 2 tablespoons olive oil
- 1 onion, finely chopped
- 3 cloves garlic, minced
- 1 tablespoon fresh ginger, grated
- 1/4 cup low-sodium soy sauce
- 1 tablespoon hoisin sauce
- 1 teaspoon rice vinegar
- 1 cup shredded carrots
- 1/4 cup chopped green onions
- 1 head butter lettuce, leaves separated
- Freshly ground black pepper

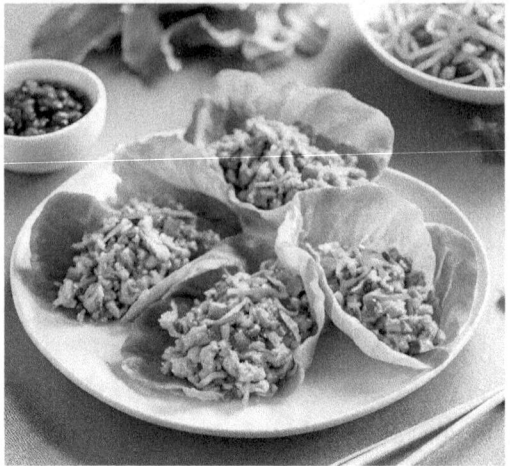

**Instructions**

1. Cook the Turkey:
   - In a large skillet, heat the olive oil over medium-high heat.
   - Add the ground turkey and cook for 5-7 minutes until browned and cooked through.
   - Add the chopped onion, minced garlic, and grated ginger. Cook for another 3-4 minutes.
2. Add the Sauces:
   - Stir in the soy sauce, hoisin sauce, rice vinegar, and freshly ground black pepper.
   - Cook for another 2-3 minutes until well combined.
3. Assemble and Serve:
   - Spoon the turkey mixture into the lettuce leaves.
   - Top with shredded carrots and chopped green onions.

**Nutrition Info (per serving)**

- Calories: 220
- Protein: 23g
- Carbohydrates: 10g
- Fiber: 3g
- Sugars: 4g
- Total Fat: 10g
- Saturated Fat: 2g
- Cholesterol: 55mg
- Sodium: 480mg

## 8. Chicken and Asparagus Skillet

**Servings:** 4
**Cooking Time:** 20 minutes

**Ingredients**

- 1 pound boneless, skinless chicken breasts, cut into strips
- 2 tablespoons olive oil
- 1 bunch asparagus, trimmed and cut into 2-inch pieces
- 1 onion, thinly sliced
- 3 cloves garlic, minced
- 1/2 cup low-sodium chicken broth
- 1 tablespoon lemon juice
- 1 teaspoon dried thyme
- Freshly ground black pepper

**Instructions**

1. Cook the Chicken:
   - In a large skillet, heat 1 tablespoon of olive oil over medium-high heat.
   - Add the chicken strips and cook for 5-7 minutes until browned and cooked through. Remove from the skillet and set aside.
2. Cook the Vegetables:
   - In the same skillet, add the remaining olive oil.
   - Add the asparagus and onion, cooking for 3-4 minutes until the vegetables are tender-crisp.
   - Add the minced garlic and cook for another 1-2 minutes.
3. Combine and Serve:
   - Return the chicken to the skillet.
   - Stir in the chicken broth, lemon juice, dried thyme, and freshly ground black pepper.
   - Cook for another 2-3 minutes until heated through and well combined.
   - Serve immediately.

**Nutrition Info (per serving)**

- Calories: 240
- Protein: 28g
- Carbohydrates: 8g
- Fiber: 3g
- Sugars: 3g
- Total Fat: 11g
- Saturated Fat: 2g
- Cholesterol: 75mg
- Sodium: 120mg

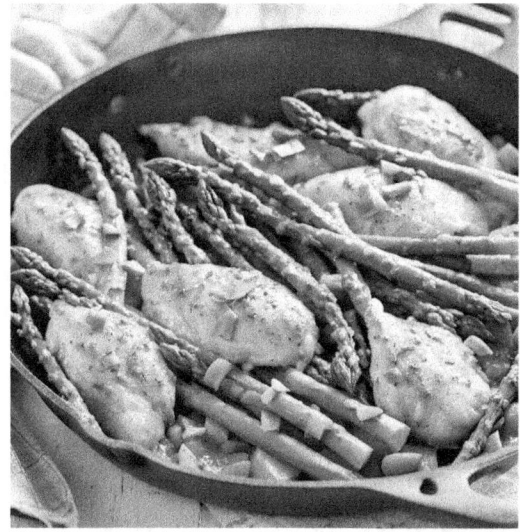

## 9. Turkey Stuffed Peppers

**Servings:** 4
**Cooking Time:** 40 minutes

**Ingredients**

- 4 large bell peppers, tops cut off and seeds removed
- 1 pound ground turkey
- 1 cup cooked quinoa
- 1 cup diced tomatoes
- 1/2 cup chopped onion
- 3 cloves garlic, minced
- 1 teaspoon ground cumin
- 1 teaspoon smoked paprika
- Freshly ground black pepper
- 1/2 cup shredded mozzarella cheese
- 1 tablespoon olive oil

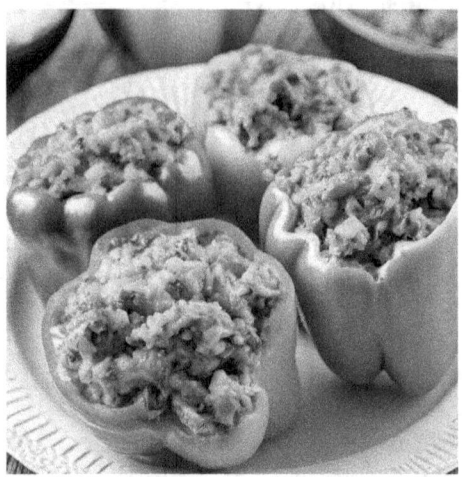

**Instructions**

1. Prepare the Filling:
   - Preheat the oven to 375°F (190°C).
   - In a large skillet, heat the olive oil over medium heat.
   - Add the ground turkey, chopped onion, and minced garlic. Cook for 5-7 minutes until the turkey is browned and cooked through.
   - Stir in the cooked quinoa, diced tomatoes, ground cumin, smoked paprika, and freshly ground black pepper. Cook for another 2-3 minutes until well combined.
2. Stuff the Peppers:
   - Place the bell peppers in a baking dish.
   - Fill each pepper with the turkey mixture and top with shredded mozzarella cheese.
3. Bake:
   - Cover with foil and bake for 30 minutes.
   - Remove the foil and bake for an additional 10 minutes until the cheese is melted and golden.
4. Serve:
   - Let cool slightly before serving.

**Nutrition Info (per serving)**

- Calories: 320   Protein: 28g   Carbohydrates: 24g
- Fiber: 5g
- Sugars: 8g
- Total Fat: 13g
- Saturated Fat: 4g
- Cholesterol: 75mg
- Sodium: 180mg

## 10. Buffalo Chicken Salad

**Servings:** 4
**Cooking Time:** 20 minutes

### Ingredients

- 1 pound boneless, skinless chicken breasts
- 1/4 cup hot sauce (like Frank's RedHot)
- 1 tablespoon olive oil
- 6 cups mixed salad greens
- 1 cup cherry tomatoes, halved
- 1/2 cup shredded carrots
- 1/2 cup chopped celery
- 1/4 cup blue cheese crumbles
- 1/4 cup plain Greek yogurt
- 2 tablespoons apple cider vinegar
- Freshly ground black pepper

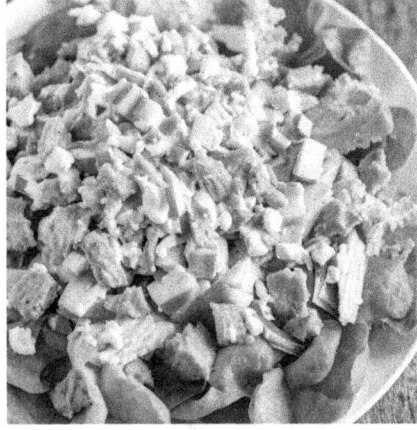

### Instructions

1. Cook the Chicken:
   - Preheat the grill or a skillet over medium-high heat.
   - Brush the chicken breasts with olive oil and grill or cook in the skillet for 6-7 minutes on each side, or until cooked through and the internal temperature reaches 165°F (75°C).
   - Remove from heat and let cool slightly before slicing.
2. Prepare the Buffalo Sauce:
   - In a bowl, toss the sliced chicken with the hot sauce.
3. Assemble the Salad:
   - In a large bowl, combine the mixed salad greens, cherry tomatoes, shredded carrots, and chopped celery.
   - Top with the buffalo chicken slices and blue cheese crumbles.
4. Prepare the Dressing:
   - In a small bowl, whisk together the Greek yogurt, apple cider vinegar, and freshly ground black pepper.
5. Serve:
   - Drizzle the dressing over the salad before serving.

### Nutrition Info (per serving)

- Calories: 300
- Protein: 30g
- Carbohydrates: 10g
- Fiber: 3g
- Sugars: 5g
- Total Fat: 16g
- Saturated Fat: 4g
- Cholesterol: 85mg
- Sodium: 420mg

## 11. Chicken Cacciatore

**Servings:** 4
**Cooking Time:** 45 minutes

**Ingredients**
- 4 boneless, skinless chicken breasts
- 2 tablespoons olive oil
- 1 onion, chopped
- 3 cloves garlic, minced
- 1 red bell pepper, chopped
- 1 green bell pepper, chopped
- 1 cup sliced mushrooms
- 1 can (14.5 ounces) diced tomatoes
- 1/2 cup low-sodium chicken broth
- 1 teaspoon dried oregano
- 1 teaspoon dried basil
- Freshly ground black pepper
- Fresh parsley (optional, for garnish)

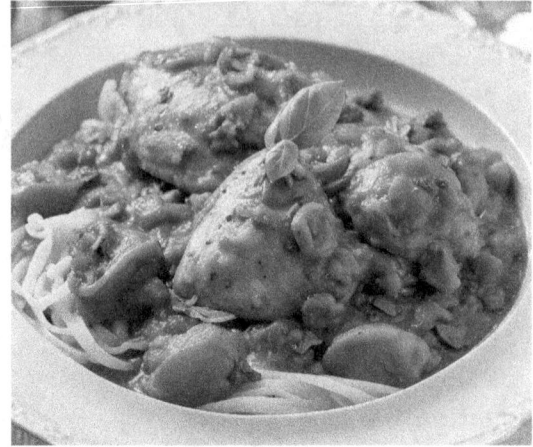

**Instructions**
1. Prepare the Chicken:
   - In a large skillet, heat the olive oil over medium-high heat.
   - Add the chicken breasts and cook for 5-7 minutes on each side until browned. Remove from the skillet and set aside.
2. Cook the Vegetables:
   - In the same skillet, add the chopped onion, minced garlic, red bell pepper, green bell pepper, and sliced mushrooms. Cook for 5-7 minutes until the vegetables are tender.
3. Combine and Simmer:
   - Return the chicken to the skillet.
   - Add the diced tomatoes, chicken broth, dried oregano, dried basil, and freshly ground black pepper.
   - Bring to a simmer, cover, and cook for 25-30 minutes until the chicken is cooked through and the sauce has thickened.
4. Serve:
   - Garnish with fresh parsley if desired.

**Nutrition Info (per serving)**
- Calories: 280   Protein: 30g
- Carbohydrates: 14g
- Fiber: 4g
- Sugars: 7g
- Total Fat: 12g
- Saturated Fat: 2g
- Cholesterol: 75mg
- Sodium: 220mg

## 12. Turkey Burgers with Sweet Potato Fries

**Servings:** 4
**Cooking Time:** 40 minutes

**Ingredients**

- 1 pound ground turkey
- 1/4 cup finely chopped onion
- 2 cloves garlic, minced
- 1 teaspoon ground cumin
- 1 teaspoon smoked paprika
- Freshly ground black pepper
- 4 whole wheat burger buns
- 2 large sweet potatoes, cut into fries
- 2 tablespoons olive oil
- 1 tablespoon fresh parsley, chopped

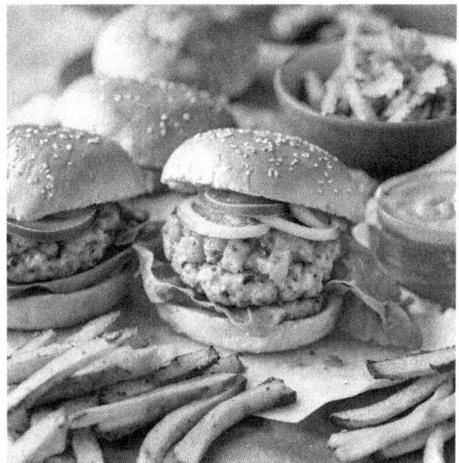

**Instructions**

1. Prepare the Sweet Potato Fries:
    - Preheat the oven to 425°F (220°C).
    - Toss the sweet potato fries with olive oil and freshly ground black pepper.
    - Spread the fries in a single layer on a baking sheet.
    - Bake for 25-30 minutes, turning halfway through, until golden and crispy.
2. Prepare the Turkey Burgers:
    - In a large bowl, combine the ground turkey, chopped onion, minced garlic, ground cumin, smoked paprika, and freshly ground black pepper. Mix until well combined.
    - Form the mixture into 4 patties.
3. Cook the Turkey Burgers:
    - Preheat a grill or skillet over medium-high heat.
    - Cook the turkey burgers for 5-7 minutes on each side until cooked through and the internal temperature reaches 165°F (75°C).
4. Assemble and Serve:
    - Place each turkey burger on a whole wheat bun.
    - Serve with sweet potato fries on the side, garnished with chopped fresh parsley.

**Nutrition Info (per serving)**

- Calories: 380
- Protein: 28g
- Carbohydrates: 45g
- Fiber: 6g
- Sugars: 8g
- Total Fat: 12g
- Saturated Fat: 2g
- Cholesterol: 75mg
- Sodium: 300mg

## 13. Chicken and Mushroom Risotto

**Servings:** 4
**Cooking Time:** 35 minutes

### Ingredients
- 1 pound boneless, skinless chicken breasts, cut into cubes
- 2 tablespoons olive oil
- 1 onion, finely chopped
- 2 cloves garlic, minced
- 1 cup Arborio rice
- 1 cup sliced mushrooms
- 4 cups low-sodium chicken broth, warmed
- 1/2 cup grated Parmesan cheese
- 1 tablespoon fresh parsley, chopped
- Freshly ground black pepper

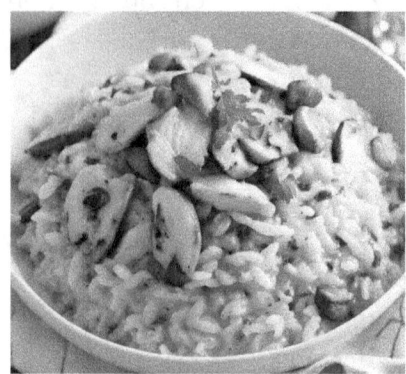

### Instructions
1. Cook the Chicken:
   - In a large skillet, heat 1 tablespoon of olive oil over medium-high heat.
   - Add the cubed chicken and cook for 5-7 minutes until browned and cooked through. Remove from the skillet and set aside.
2. Cook the Vegetables:
   - In the same skillet, add the remaining olive oil.
   - Add the chopped onion and cook for 3-4 minutes until softened.
   - Add the minced garlic and sliced mushrooms, cooking for another 3-4 minutes.
3. Prepare the Risotto:
   - Stir in the Arborio rice and cook for 2 minutes until lightly toasted.
   - Add one ladleful of warm chicken broth to the rice mixture, stirring until the liquid is absorbed.
   - Continue adding the broth one ladleful at a time, stirring frequently, until the rice is creamy and tender, about 18-20 minutes.
4. Combine and Serve:
   - Stir in the cooked chicken, grated Parmesan cheese, and freshly ground black pepper.
   - Garnish with chopped fresh parsley before serving.

### Nutrition Info (per serving)
- Calories: 350   Protein: 28g   Carbohydrates: 40g
- Fiber: 2g
- Sugars: 3g
- Total Fat: 10g
- Saturated Fat: 3g
- Cholesterol: 75mg
- Sodium: 320mg

## 14. Grilled Turkey Kebabs

**Servings:** 4
**Cooking Time:** 20 minutes

**Ingredients**
- 1 pound turkey breast, cut into 1-inch cubes
- 2 tablespoons olive oil
- 1 tablespoon lemon juice
- 2 cloves garlic, minced
- 1 teaspoon dried oregano
- Freshly ground black pepper
- 1 red bell pepper, cut into 1-inch pieces
- 1 yellow bell pepper, cut into 1-inch pieces
- 1 red onion, cut into wedges
- Skewers

**Instructions**
1. Prepare the Marinade:
   - In a bowl, mix the olive oil, lemon juice, minced garlic, dried oregano, and freshly ground black pepper.
   - Add the turkey cubes and marinate for at least 30 minutes.
2. Assemble the Kebabs:
   - Thread the marinated turkey, red bell pepper, yellow bell pepper, and red onion onto skewers.
3. Grill the Kebabs:
   - Preheat the grill to medium-high heat.
   - Grill the kebabs for 10-12 minutes, turning occasionally, until the turkey is cooked through and the vegetables are tender.
4. Serve:
   - Serve the kebabs immediately.

**Nutrition Info (per serving)**
- Calories: 280
- Protein: 30g
- Carbohydrates: 10g
- Fiber: 2g
- Sugars: 5g
- Total Fat: 14g
- Saturated Fat: 2.5g
- Cholesterol: 75mg
- Sodium: 150mg

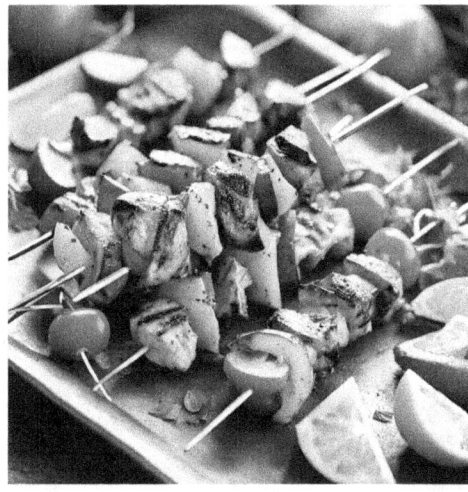

## 15. Slow Cooker Chicken Tikka Masala

**Servings: 4**
**Cooking Time: 6 hours**
**Ingredients**

- 1 pound boneless, skinless chicken thighs, cut into chunks
- 1 onion, chopped
- 3 cloves garlic, minced
- 1 tablespoon fresh ginger, grated
- 1 can (14.5 ounces) diced tomatoes
- 1 cup coconut milk
- 2 tablespoons tomato paste
- 2 teaspoons ground cumin
- 2 teaspoons ground coriander
- 1 teaspoon ground turmeric
- 1 teaspoon garam masala
- Freshly ground black pepper
- 1 tablespoon olive oil
- Fresh cilantro (optional, for garnish)

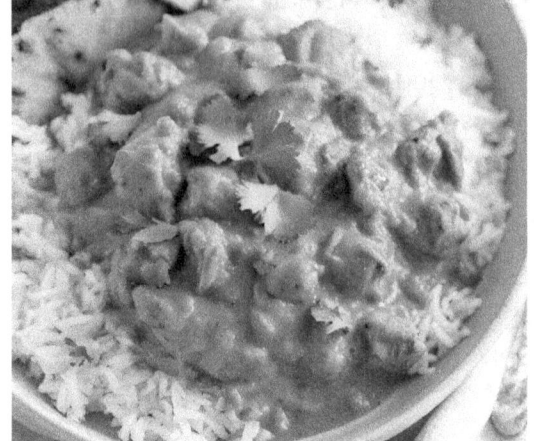

**Instructions**

1. Prepare the Ingredients:
    - In a large skillet, heat the olive oil over medium heat.
    - Add the chopped onion, minced garlic, and grated ginger. Cook for 3-4 minutes until softened.
2. Combine in Slow Cooker:
    - Transfer the onion mixture to the slow cooker.
    - Add the chicken chunks, diced tomatoes, coconut milk, tomato paste, ground cumin, ground coriander, ground turmeric, garam masala, and freshly ground black pepper.
    - Stir to combine.
3. Cook:
    - Cover and cook on low for 6 hours, or until the chicken is tender and the flavors are well combined.
4. Serve:
    - Garnish with fresh cilantro if desired.
    - Serve with cooked rice or naan bread.

**Nutrition Info (per serving)**

- Calories: 360   Protein: 28g   Carbohydrates: 14g   Fiber: 4g
- Sugars: 6g   Total Fat: 20g   Saturated Fat: 10g
- Cholesterol: 110mg
- Sodium: 220mg

## 16. Greek Chicken Bowls

**Servings:** 4
**Cooking Time:** 30 minutes

**Ingredients**

- 1 pound boneless, skinless chicken breasts, cut into cubes
- 2 tablespoons olive oil
- 1 teaspoon dried oregano
- 1 teaspoon garlic powder
- Freshly ground black pepper
- 1 cup quinoa, cooked
- 1 cup cherry tomatoes, halved
- 1 cucumber, diced
- 1/4 cup red onion, finely chopped
- 1/4 cup Kalamata olives, sliced
- 1/4 cup feta cheese, crumbled
- 2 tablespoons lemon juice
- Fresh parsley (optional, for garnish)

**Instructions**

1. Prepare the Chicken:
   - In a large skillet, heat the olive oil over medium-high heat.
   - Add the chicken cubes, dried oregano, garlic powder, and freshly ground black pepper. Cook for 7-10 minutes until the chicken is browned and cooked through.
2. Prepare the Bowls:
   - Divide the cooked quinoa among four bowls.
   - Top each bowl with the cooked chicken, cherry tomatoes, cucumber, red onion, Kalamata olives, and feta cheese.
3. Serve:
   - Drizzle with lemon juice and garnish with fresh parsley if desired.

**Nutrition Info (per serving)**

- Calories: 360
- Protein: 28g
- Carbohydrates: 32g
- Fiber: 6g
- Sugars: 5g
- Total Fat: 15g
- Saturated Fat: 4g
- Cholesterol: 75mg
- Sodium: 300mg

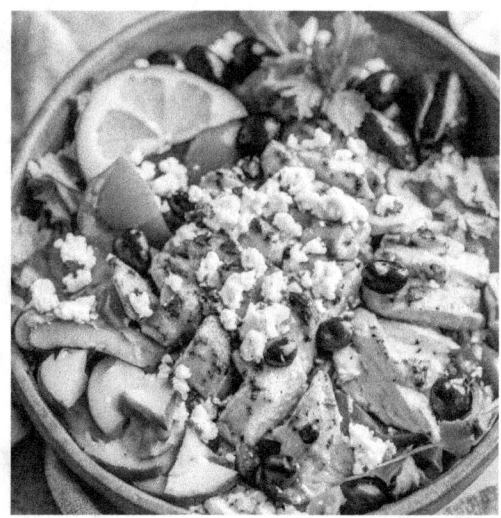

## 17. Honey Mustard Chicken Thighs

**Servings:** 4
**Cooking Time:** 40 minutes

### Ingredients
- 8 boneless, skinless chicken thighs
- 1/4 cup honey
- 1/4 cup Dijon mustard
- 2 tablespoons olive oil
- 1 teaspoon dried thyme
- Freshly ground black pepper
- Fresh parsley (optional, for garnish)

### Instructions
1. Preheat Oven:
   - Preheat your oven to 375°F (190°C).
2. Prepare the Sauce:
   - In a bowl, whisk together the honey, Dijon mustard, olive oil, dried thyme, and freshly ground black pepper.
3. Bake the Chicken:
   - Place the chicken thighs in a baking dish.
   - Pour the honey mustard sauce over the chicken, making sure each piece is well coated.
   - Bake for 35-40 minutes, or until the chicken is cooked through and the internal temperature reaches 165°F (75°C).
4. Serve:
   - Garnish with fresh parsley if desired.

### Nutrition Info (per serving)
- Calories: 380
- Protein: 28g
- Carbohydrates: 14g
- Fiber: 1g
- Sugars: 12g
- Total Fat: 22g
- Saturated Fat: 5g
- Cholesterol: 115mg
- Sodium: 240mg

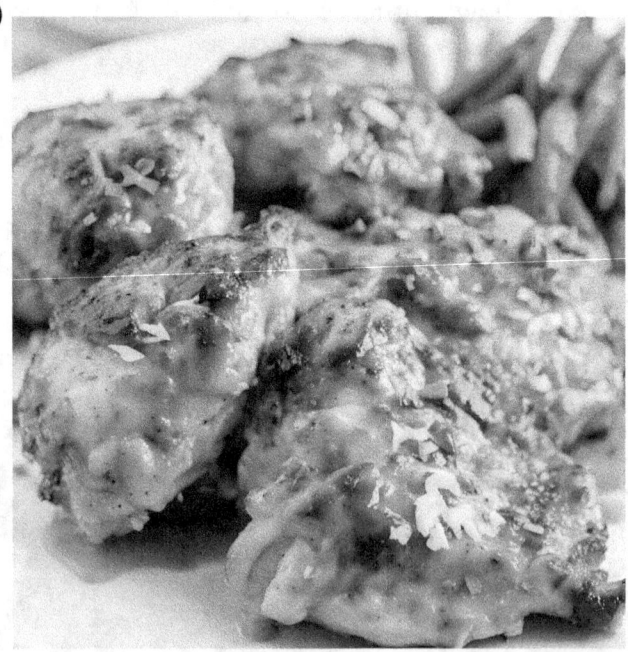

## 18. Pulled Turkey Tacos

**Servings:** 4
**Cooking Time:** 6 hours

**Ingredients**
- 1 pound turkey breast
- 1 onion, sliced
- 3 cloves garlic, minced
- 1 cup low-sodium chicken broth
- 1 teaspoon ground cumin
- 1 teaspoon chili powder
- Freshly ground black pepper
- 8 small corn tortillas
- 1 cup shredded lettuce
- 1/2 cup diced tomatoes
- 1/4 cup chopped cilantro
- 1 lime, cut into wedges

**Instructions**

1. Prepare the Turkey:
   - Place the turkey breast in a slow cooker.
   - Add the sliced onion, minced garlic, chicken broth, ground cumin, chili powder, and freshly ground black pepper.
   - Cover and cook on low for 6 hours, or until the turkey is tender and easily shredded.
2. Shred the Turkey:
   - Remove the turkey from the slow cooker and shred with two forks.
   - Return the shredded turkey to the slow cooker and mix with the cooking juices.
3. Assemble the Tacos:
   - Warm the corn tortillas in a skillet or microwave.
   - Fill each tortilla with the pulled turkey, shredded lettuce, diced tomatoes, and chopped cilantro.
4. Serve:
   - Serve with lime wedges.

**Nutrition Info (per serving)**
- Calories: 300
- Protein: 30g
- Carbohydrates: 30g
- Fiber: 5g
- Sugars: 3g
- Total Fat: 8g
- Saturated Fat: 2g
- Cholesterol: 70mg
- Sodium: 180mg

## 19. Balsamic Chicken and Vegetables

**Servings:** 4
**Cooking Time:** 30 minutes

**Ingredients**

- 4 boneless, skinless chicken breasts
- 2 tablespoons olive oil
- 1/4 cup balsamic vinegar
- 1 tablespoon honey
- 1 teaspoon dried basil
- Freshly ground black pepper
- 1 red bell pepper, sliced
- 1 yellow bell pepper, sliced
- 1 zucchini, sliced
- 1 red onion, sliced
- Fresh basil (optional, for garnish)

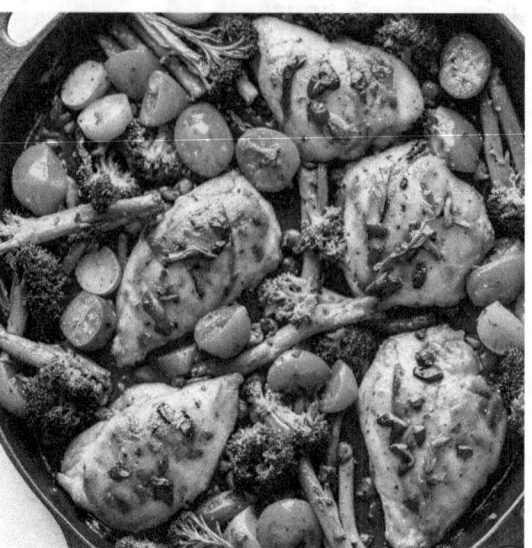

**Instructions**

1. Prepare the Marinade:
   - In a bowl, whisk together the balsamic vinegar, honey, olive oil, dried basil, and freshly ground black pepper.
2. Marinate the Chicken:
   - Place the chicken breasts in a shallow dish and pour half of the balsamic marinade over them.
   - Marinate for at least 30 minutes.
3. Cook the Chicken:
   - Preheat a grill or skillet over medium-high heat.
   - Grill or cook the chicken for 6-7 minutes on each side, or until cooked through and the internal temperature reaches 165°F (75°C).
4. Cook the Vegetables:
   - In a large skillet, heat 1 tablespoon of olive oil over medium-high heat.
   - Add the sliced bell peppers, zucchini, and red onion.
   - Cook for 5-7 minutes until tender-crisp.
   - Pour the remaining balsamic marinade over the vegetables and cook for another 2-3 minutes.
5. Serve:
   - Serve the chicken with the balsamic vegetables and garnish with fresh basil if desired.

**Nutrition Info (per serving)**

- Calories: 320   Protein: 28g   Carbohydrates: 18g   Fiber: 4g
- Sugars: 10g   Total Fat: 14g   Saturated Fat: 2.5g
- Cholesterol: 75mg
- Sodium: 180mg

## 20. Barbecue Chicken Pizza

**Servings:** 4
**Cooking Time:** 25 minutes

**Ingredients**
- 1 pre-made whole wheat pizza crust
- 1/2 cup barbecue sauce
- 1 pound boneless, skinless chicken breasts, cooked and shredded
- 1/2 red onion, thinly sliced
- 1 cup shredded mozzarella cheese
- 1/4 cup chopped fresh cilantro

**Instructions**
1. Preheat Oven:
   - Preheat your oven to 425°F (220°C).
2. Prepare the Chicken:
   - In a bowl, toss the shredded chicken with 1/4 cup of the barbecue sauce.
3. Assemble the Pizza:
   - Place the whole wheat pizza crust on a baking sheet.
   - Spread the remaining 1/4 cup of barbecue sauce evenly over the crust.
   - Top with the shredded barbecue chicken, thinly sliced red onion, and shredded mozzarella cheese.
4. Bake:
   - Bake in the preheated oven for 12-15 minutes, or until the cheese is melted and bubbly.
5. Serve:
   - Garnish with chopped fresh cilantro before serving.

**Nutrition Info (per serving)**
- Calories: 380
- Protein: 30g
- Carbohydrates: 42g
- Fiber: 5g
- Sugars: 12g
- Total Fat: 12g
- Saturated Fat: 5g
- Cholesterol: 75mg
- Sodium: 520mg

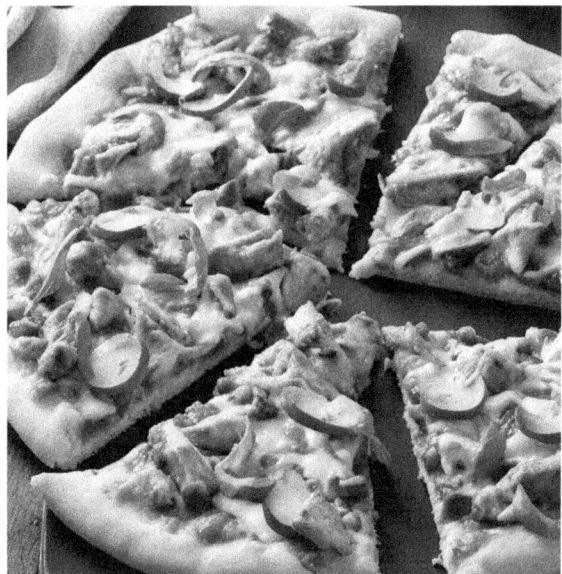

## 21. Turkey Sloppy Joes

**Servings:** 4
**Cooking Time:** 30 minutes

**Ingredients**
- 1 pound ground turkey
- 1 onion, finely chopped
- 2 cloves garlic, minced
- 1 green bell pepper, chopped
- 1 cup tomato sauce
- 1/4 cup tomato paste
- 1 tablespoon Worcestershire sauce
- 1 tablespoon Dijon mustard
- 1 tablespoon honey
- Freshly ground black pepper
- 4 whole wheat buns

**Instructions**
1. Cook the Turkey:
   - In a large skillet, heat a tablespoon of olive oil over medium heat.
   - Add the ground turkey, chopped onion, minced garlic, and chopped green bell pepper. Cook for 7-10 minutes until the turkey is browned and the vegetables are tender.
2. Prepare the Sauce:
   - Stir in the tomato sauce, tomato paste, Worcestershire sauce, Dijon mustard, honey, and freshly ground black pepper.
   - Reduce the heat and simmer for 10-15 minutes until the mixture thickens.
3. Serve:
   - Spoon the turkey mixture onto whole wheat buns and serve immediately.

**Nutrition Info (per serving)**
- Calories: 340
- Protein: 28g
- Carbohydrates: 35g
- Fiber: 6g
- Sugars: 10g
- Total Fat: 12g
- Saturated Fat: 2.5g
- Cholesterol: 70mg
- Sodium: 440mg

## 22. Chicken and Spinach Stuffed Shells
**Servings:** 4
**Cooking Time:** 40 minutes
**Ingredients**
- 12 large pasta shells
- 1 pound boneless, skinless chicken breasts, cooked and shredded
- 2 cups fresh spinach, chopped
- 1 cup ricotta cheese
- 1/2 cup grated Parmesan cheese
- 1 egg, beaten
- 2 cups marinara sauce
- Freshly ground black pepper

**Instructions**
1. Preheat Oven:
    - Preheat your oven to 375°F (190°C).
2. Prepare the Filling:
    - In a large bowl, combine the shredded chicken, chopped spinach, ricotta cheese, grated Parmesan cheese, beaten egg, and freshly ground black pepper.
3. Cook the Pasta:
    - Cook the pasta shells according to package instructions until al dente. Drain and let cool slightly.
4. Stuff the Shells:
    - Fill each pasta shell with the chicken and spinach mixture.
    - Spread 1 cup of marinara sauce on the bottom of a baking dish.
    - Place the stuffed shells in the dish and cover with the remaining marinara sauce.
5. Bake:
    - Cover with foil and bake for 25-30 minutes, or until the filling is hot and the sauce is bubbly.

**Nutrition Info (per serving)**
- Calories: 380
- Protein: 32g
- Carbohydrates: 34g
- Fiber: 5g
- Sugars: 8g
- Total Fat: 14g
- Saturated Fat: 6g
- Cholesterol: 110mg
- Sodium: 520mg

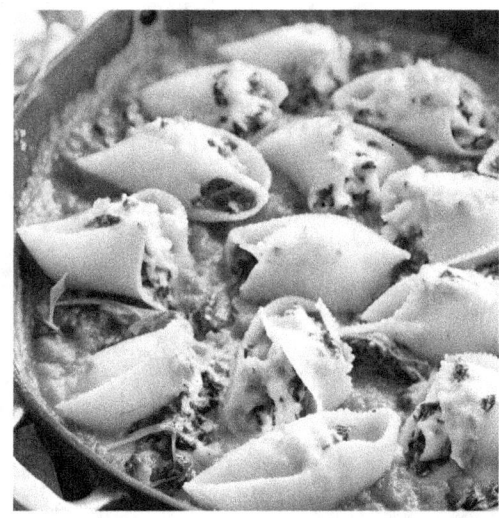

## 23. Lemon Garlic Turkey Breast

**Servings:** 4
**Cooking Time:** 1 hour 30 minutes

**Ingredients**
- 1 turkey breast (about 3 pounds)
- 1/4 cup olive oil
- 4 cloves garlic, minced
- 2 tablespoons lemon juice
- 1 tablespoon lemon zest
- 1 teaspoon dried thyme
- Freshly ground black pepper
- Lemon wedges (for serving)

**Instructions**

1. Preheat Oven:
   - Preheat your oven to 375°F (190°C).
2. Prepare the Turkey:
   - In a small bowl, mix the olive oil, minced garlic, lemon juice, lemon zest, dried thyme, and freshly ground black pepper.
   - Rub the mixture all over the turkey breast, including under the skin.
3. Roast the Turkey:
   - Place the turkey breast on a rack in a roasting pan.
   - Roast for 1 hour 20 minutes to 1 hour 30 minutes, or until the internal temperature reaches 165°F (75°C).
   - Let rest for 10 minutes before slicing.
4. Serve:
   - Serve with lemon wedges.

**Nutrition Info (per serving)**
- Calories: 380
- Protein: 52g
- Carbohydrates: 2g
- Fiber: 0g
- Sugars: 0g
- Total Fat: 18g
- Saturated Fat: 3g
- Cholesterol: 140mg
- Sodium: 120mg

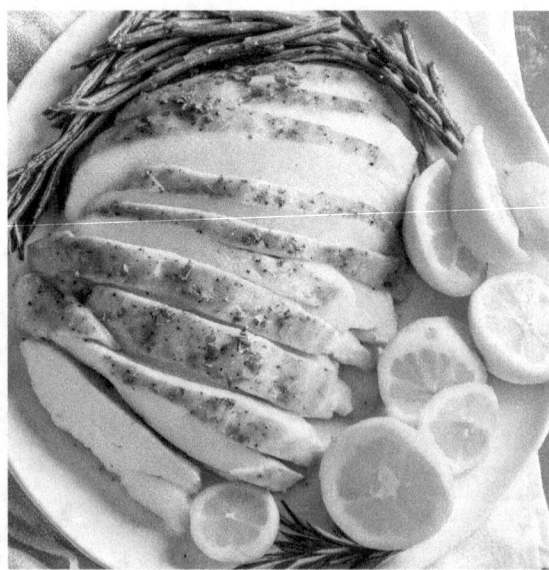

## 24. Chicken Paillard

**Servings:** 4
**Cooking Time:** 20 minutes
**Ingredients**
- 4 boneless, skinless chicken breasts
- 2 tablespoons olive oil
- 1 tablespoon lemon juice
- 1 teaspoon dried oregano
- 1 teaspoon garlic powder
- Freshly ground black pepper
- Mixed greens (for serving)
- Cherry tomatoes (for serving)
- Lemon wedges (for serving)

**Instructions**
1. Prepare the Chicken:
   - Place the chicken breasts between two pieces of plastic wrap and pound to an even thickness.
   - In a bowl, mix the olive oil, lemon juice, dried oregano, garlic powder, and freshly ground black pepper.
   - Rub the mixture all over the chicken breasts.
2. Cook the Chicken:
   - Heat a large skillet over medium-high heat.
   - Cook the chicken breasts for 4-5 minutes on each side, or until cooked through and the internal temperature reaches 165°F (75°C).
3. Serve:
   - Serve the chicken paillard over mixed greens and cherry tomatoes, with lemon wedges on the side.

**Nutrition Info (per serving)**
- Calories: 260
- Protein: 30g
- Carbohydrates: 3g
- Fiber: 1g
- Sugars: 1g
- Total Fat: 14g
- Saturated Fat: 2.5g
- Cholesterol: 80mg
- Sodium: 110mg

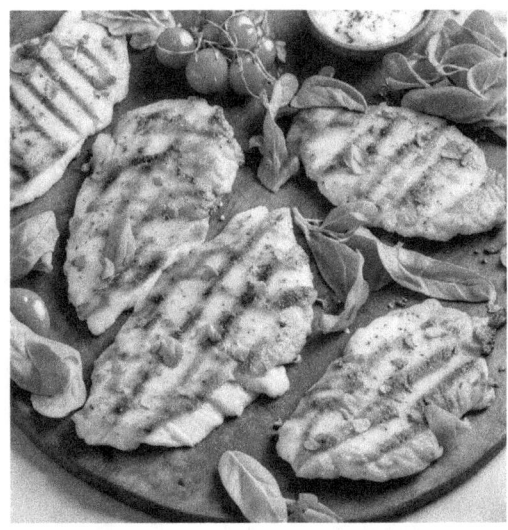

## 25. Turkey Meatloaf

**Servings:** 4
**Cooking Time:** 1 hour

**Ingredients**

- 1 pound ground turkey
- 1/2 cup finely chopped onion
- 2 cloves garlic, minced
- 1/2 cup whole wheat bread crumbs
- 1 egg, beaten
- 1/4 cup tomato sauce
- 1 tablespoon Worcestershire sauce
- 1 teaspoon dried thyme
- Freshly ground black pepper
- 1/4 cup ketchup

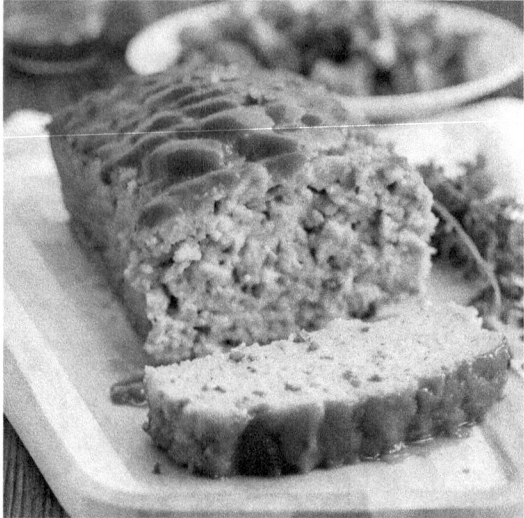

**Instructions**

1. Preheat Oven:
   - Preheat your oven to 350°F (175°C).
2. Prepare the Meatloaf:
   - In a large bowl, combine the ground turkey, chopped onion, minced garlic, bread crumbs, beaten egg, tomato sauce, Worcestershire sauce, dried thyme, and freshly ground black pepper. Mix until well combined.
3. Shape the Meatloaf:
   - Transfer the mixture to a loaf pan and shape into a loaf.
   - Spread the ketchup over the top of the meatloaf.
4. Bake:
   - Bake for 50-60 minutes, or until the internal temperature reaches 165°F (75°C).
   - Let rest for 10 minutes before slicing.

**Nutrition Info (per serving)**

- Calories: 300
- Protein: 28g
- Carbohydrates: 16g
- Fiber: 2g
- Sugars: 6g
- Total Fat: 14g
- Saturated Fat: 3.5g
- Cholesterol: 110mg
- Sodium: 400mg

# 10-WEEK MEAL PLAN

## Week 1
Monday
- Breakfast: Avocado Toast with Poached Egg
- Lunch: Turkey and Spinach Meatballs
- Dinner: Grilled Chicken with Avocado Salsa

Tuesday
- Breakfast: Quinoa Porridge
- Lunch: Spinach and Feta Wrap
- Dinner: Lemon Herb Roasted Chicken

Wednesday
- Breakfast: Oatmeal with Mixed Berries
- Lunch: Greek Chicken Bowls
- Dinner: Chicken Stir-Fry with Broccoli

Thursday
- Breakfast: Smoothie Bowl
- Lunch: Turkey Sloppy Joes
- Dinner: Chicken and Mushroom Risotto

Friday
- Breakfast: Vegetable Omelet
- Lunch: Baked Pesto Chicken
- Dinner: Pulled Turkey Tacos

Saturday
- Breakfast: Banana Pancakes
- Lunch: Grilled Turkey Kebabs
- Dinner: Balsamic Chicken and Vegetables

Sunday
- Breakfast: Sweet Potato Hash
- Lunch: Chicken Cacciatore
- Dinner: Turkey Stuffed Peppers

## Week 2
Monday
- Breakfast: Nutty Rice Pudding
- Lunch: Barbecue Chicken Pizza
- Dinner: Chicken Paillard

Tuesday
- Breakfast: Buckwheat Crepes
- Lunch: Lemon Garlic Turkey Breast
- Dinner: Turkey Meatloaf

Wednesday
- Breakfast: Muesli and Yogurt
- Lunch: Chicken and Spinach Stuffed Shells
- Dinner: Smoked Paprika Chicken

Thursday
- Breakfast: Spinach and Feta Wrap
- Lunch: Turkey Burgers with Sweet Potato Fries
- Dinner: Chicken and Asparagus Skillet

Friday
- Breakfast: Almond Butter and Banana Sandwich
- Lunch: Chicken Stir-Fry with Broccoli
- Dinner: Slow Cooker Chicken Tikka Masala

Saturday
- Breakfast: Egg Muffins
- Lunch: Turkey Sloppy Joes
- Dinner: Greek Chicken Bowls

Sunday
- Breakfast: Tofu Scramble
- Lunch: Honey Mustard Chicken Thighs
- Dinner: Lemon Garlic Turkey Breast

## Week 3

Monday
- Breakfast: Pumpkin Oatmeal
- Lunch: Grilled Chicken with Avocado Salsa
- Dinner: Turkey and Spinach Meatballs

Tuesday
- Breakfast: Turkey Sausage and Veggie Skillet
- Lunch: Asian Turkey Lettuce Wraps
- Dinner: Balsamic Chicken and Vegetables

Wednesday
- Breakfast: Ricotta and Tomato Toast
- Lunch: Chicken Paillard
- Dinner: Pulled Turkey Tacos

Thursday
- Breakfast: Breakfast Lentils
- Lunch: Barbecue Chicken Pizza
- Dinner: Chicken and Mushroom Risotto

Friday
- Breakfast: Mango and Coconut Rice
- Lunch: Lemon Herb Roasted Chicken
- Dinner: Greek Chicken Bowls

Saturday
- Breakfast: Savory Porridge
- Lunch: Turkey Stuffed Peppers
- Dinner: Grilled Turkey Kebabs

Sunday
- Breakfast: Stuffed Breakfast Peppers
- Lunch: Chicken Cacciatore
- Dinner: Chicken and Spinach Stuffed Shells

# Week 4

Monday
- Breakfast: Apple-Cinnamon Oat Bake
- Lunch: Baked Pesto Chicken
- Dinner: Chicken Stir-Fry with Broccoli

Tuesday
- Breakfast: Almond Flour Waffles
- Lunch: Smoked Paprika Chicken
- Dinner: Slow Cooker Chicken Tikka Masala

Wednesday
- Breakfast: Zucchini and Onion Frittata
- Lunch: Chicken Paillard
- Dinner: Lemon Garlic Turkey Breast

Thursday
- Breakfast: Shakshuka
- Lunch: Greek Chicken Bowls
- Dinner: Honey Mustard Chicken Thighs

Friday
- Breakfast: Curried Lentils with Spinach
- Lunch: Turkey Burgers with Sweet Potato Fries
- Dinner: Barbecue Chicken Pizza

Saturday
- Breakfast: Mushroom Stroganoff
- Lunch: Chicken and Asparagus Skillet
- Dinner: Turkey Meatloaf

Sunday
- Breakfast: Garlic Green Beans
- Lunch: Chicken Cacciatore
- Dinner: Turkey and Spinach Meatballs

# Week 5
Monday
- Breakfast: Vegetable Stir-Fry with Tofu
- Lunch: Balsamic Chicken and Vegetables
- Dinner: Pulled Turkey Tacos

Tuesday
- Breakfast: Tomato Gazpacho
- Lunch: Greek Chicken Bowls
- Dinner: Chicken and Mushroom Risotto

Wednesday
- Breakfast: Cabbage Slaw with Sesame Dressing
- Lunch: Honey Mustard Chicken Thighs
- Dinner: Grilled Turkey Kebabs

Thursday
- Breakfast: Roasted Turnips with Rosemary
- Lunch: Turkey Sloppy Joes
- Dinner: Smoked Paprika Chicken

Friday
- Breakfast: Sautéed Swiss Chard with Pine Nuts
- Lunch: Chicken Stir-Fry with Broccoli
- Dinner: Chicken and Spinach Stuffed Shells

Saturday
- Breakfast: Vegan Ratatouille
- Lunch: Barbecue Chicken Pizza
- Dinner: Slow Cooker Chicken Tikka Masala

Sunday
- Breakfast: Spinach and Feta Pie
- Lunch: Chicken Paillard
- Dinner: Turkey Meatloaf

# Week 6
Monday
- Breakfast: Avocado Toast with Poached Egg
- Lunch: Grilled Salmon with Dill Yogurt Sauce
- Dinner: Turkey and Spinach Meatballs

Tuesday
- Breakfast: Quinoa Porridge
- Lunch: Spinach and Feta Wrap
- Dinner: Lemon Herb Roasted Chicken

Wednesday
- Breakfast: Oatmeal with Mixed Berries
- Lunch: Greek Chicken Bowls
- Dinner: Chicken Stir-Fry with Broccoli

Thursday
- Breakfast: Smoothie Bowl
- Lunch: Turkey Sloppy Joes
- Dinner: Chicken and Mushroom Risotto

Friday
- Breakfast: Vegetable Omelet
- Lunch: Baked Pesto Chicken
- Dinner: Pulled Turkey Tacos

Saturday
- Breakfast: Banana Pancakes
- Lunch: Grilled Turkey Kebabs
- Dinner: Balsamic Chicken and Vegetables

Sunday
- Breakfast: Sweet Potato Hash
- Lunch: Chicken Cacciatore
- Dinner: Turkey Stuffed Peppers

# Week 7

Monday
- Breakfast: Nutty Rice Pudding
- Lunch: Barbecue Chicken Pizza
- Dinner: Chicken Paillard

Tuesday
- Breakfast: Buckwheat Crepes
- Lunch: Lemon Garlic Turkey Breast
- Dinner: Turkey Meatloaf

Wednesday
- Breakfast: Muesli and Yogurt
- Lunch: Chicken and Spinach Stuffed Shells
- Dinner: Smoked Paprika Chicken

Thursday
- Breakfast: Spinach and Feta Wrap
- Lunch: Turkey Burgers with Sweet Potato Fries
- Dinner: Chicken and Asparagus Skillet

Friday
- Breakfast: Almond Butter and Banana Sandwich
- Lunch: Chicken Stir-Fry with Broccoli
- Dinner: Slow Cooker Chicken Tikka Masala

Saturday
- Breakfast: Egg Muffins
- Lunch: Turkey Sloppy Joes
- Dinner: Greek Chicken Bowls

Sunday
- Breakfast: Tofu Scramble
- Lunch: Honey Mustard Chicken Thighs
- Dinner: Lemon Garlic Turkey Breast

## Week 8

Monday
- Breakfast: Pumpkin Oatmeal
- Lunch: Grilled Chicken with Avocado Salsa
- Dinner: Turkey and Spinach Meatballs

Tuesday
- Breakfast: Turkey Sausage and Veggie Skillet
- Lunch: Asian Turkey Lettuce Wraps
- Dinner: Balsamic Chicken and Vegetables

Wednesday
- Breakfast: Ricotta and Tomato Toast
- Lunch: Chicken Paillard
- Dinner: Pulled Turkey Tacos

Thursday
- Breakfast: Breakfast Lentils
- Lunch: Barbecue Chicken Pizza
- Dinner: Chicken and Mushroom Risotto

Friday
- Breakfast: Mango and Coconut Rice
- Lunch: Lemon Herb Roasted Chicken
- Dinner: Greek Chicken Bowls

Saturday
- Breakfast: Savory Porridge
- Lunch: Turkey Stuffed Peppers
- Dinner: Grilled Turkey Kebabs

Sunday
- Breakfast: Stuffed Breakfast Peppers
- Lunch: Chicken Cacciatore
- Dinner: Chicken and Spinach Stuffed Shells

# Week 9
Monday
- Breakfast: Apple-Cinnamon Oat Bake
- Lunch: Baked Pesto Chicken
- Dinner: Chicken Stir-Fry with Broccoli

Tuesday
- Breakfast: Almond Flour Waffles
- Lunch: Smoked Paprika Chicken
- Dinner: Slow Cooker Chicken Tikka Masala

Wednesday
- Breakfast: Zucchini and Onion Frittata
- Lunch: Chicken Paillard
- Dinner: Lemon Garlic Turkey Breast

Thursday
- Breakfast: Shakshuka
- Lunch: Greek Chicken Bowls
- Dinner: Honey Mustard Chicken Thighs

Friday
- Breakfast: Curried Lentils with Spinach
- Lunch: Turkey Burgers with Sweet Potato Fries
- Dinner: Barbecue Chicken Pizza

Saturday
- Breakfast: Mushroom Stroganoff
- Lunch: Chicken and Asparagus Skillet
- Dinner: Turkey Meatloaf

Sunday
- Breakfast: Garlic Green Beans
- Lunch: Chicken Cacciatore
- Dinner: Turkey and Spinach Meatballs

# Week 10
Monday
- Breakfast: Vegetable Stir-Fry with Tofu
- Lunch: Balsamic Chicken and Vegetables
- Dinner: Pulled Turkey Tacos

Tuesday
- Breakfast: Tomato Gazpacho
- Lunch: Greek Chicken Bowls
- Dinner: Chicken and Mushroom Risotto

Wednesday
- Breakfast: Cabbage Slaw with Sesame Dressing
- Lunch: Honey Mustard Chicken Thighs
- Dinner: Grilled Turkey Kebabs

Thursday
- Breakfast: Roasted Turnips with Rosemary
- Lunch: Turkey Sloppy Joes
- Dinner: Smoked Paprika Chicken

Friday
- Breakfast: Sautéed Swiss Chard with Pine Nuts
- Lunch: Chicken Stir-Fry with Broccoli
- Dinner: Chicken and Spinach Stuffed Shells

Saturday
- Breakfast: Vegan Ratatouille
- Lunch: Barbecue Chicken Pizza
- Dinner: Slow Cooker Chicken Tikka Masala

Sunday
- Breakfast: Spinach and Feta Pie
- Lunch: Chicken Paillard
- Dinner: Turkey Meatloaf

This additional 5-week meal pl

# Weekly Meal planner + Journal

|     | BREAKFAST | LUNCH | DINNER | SNACKS |
|-----|-----------|-------|--------|--------|
| MON |           |       |        |        |
| TUE |           |       |        |        |
| WED |           |       |        |        |
| THU |           |       |        |        |
| FRI |           |       |        |        |
| SAT |           |       |        |        |
| SUN |           |       |        |        |

What are your primary health goals and expectations in starting the Peripheral Neuropathy Diet?

..............................................................................................................................................................................

..............................................................................................................................................................................

..............................................................................................................................................................................

..............................................................................................................................................................................

..............................................................................................................................................................................

..............................................................................................................................................................................

# Weekly Meal planner + Journal

|  | BREAKFAST | LUNCH | DINNER | SNACKS |
|---|---|---|---|---|
| MON |  |  |  |  |
| TUE |  |  |  |  |
| WED |  |  |  |  |
| THU |  |  |  |  |
| FRI |  |  |  |  |
| SAT |  |  |  |  |
| SUN |  |  |  |  |

How would you describe your current eating habits? What changes do you anticipate making with this new diet?

..................................................................................................................................................
..................................................................................................................................................
..................................................................................................................................................
..................................................................................................................................................
..................................................................................................................................................
..................................................................................................................................................
..................................................................................................................................................

# Weekly Meal planner + Journal

|     | BREAKFAST | LUNCH | DINNER | SNACKS |
|-----|-----------|-------|--------|--------|
| MON |           |       |        |        |
| TUE |           |       |        |        |
| WED |           |       |        |        |
| THU |           |       |        |        |
| FRI |           |       |        |        |
| SAT |           |       |        |        |
| SUN |           |       |        |        |

Which symptoms of peripheral neuropathy are you currently experiencing? How do you hope they will change with this diet?

..........................................................................................................................................................................................

..........................................................................................................................................................................................

..........................................................................................................................................................................................

..........................................................................................................................................................................................

..........................................................................................................................................................................................

..........................................................................................................................................................................................

..........................................................................................................................................................................................

# Weekly Meal planner + Journal

|     | BREAKFAST | LUNCH | DINNER | SNACKS |
|-----|-----------|-------|--------|--------|
| MON |           |       |        |        |
| TUE |           |       |        |        |
| WED |           |       |        |        |
| THU |           |       |        |        |
| FRI |           |       |        |        |
| SAT |           |       |        |        |
| SUN |           |       |        |        |

**Are there any specific foods that you believe worsen your symptoms? How do you plan to avoid these foods?**

.................................................................................................................................................................
.................................................................................................................................................................
.................................................................................................................................................................
.................................................................................................................................................................
.................................................................................................................................................................
.................................................................................................................................................................
.................................................................................................................................................................

# Weekly Meal planner + Journal

|     | BREAKFAST | LUNCH | DINNER | SNACKS |
|-----|-----------|-------|--------|--------|
| MON |           |       |        |        |
| TUE |           |       |        |        |
| WED |           |       |        |        |
| THU |           |       |        |        |
| FRI |           |       |        |        |
| SAT |           |       |        |        |
| SUN |           |       |        |        |

How comfortable are you with meal planning? What strategies can you use to ensure you stick to the diet?

..............................................................................................................................................................................

..............................................................................................................................................................................

..............................................................................................................................................................................

..............................................................................................................................................................................

..............................................................................................................................................................................

..............................................................................................................................................................................

..............................................................................................................................................................................

# Weekly Meal planner + Journal

|  | BREAKFAST | LUNCH | DINNER | SNACKS |
|---|---|---|---|---|
| MON | | | | |
| TUE | | | | |
| WED | | | | |
| THU | | | | |
| FRI | | | | |
| SAT | | | | |
| SUN | | | | |

What is your current level of cooking skills? Are there any new recipes or cooking techniques you are excited to try?

...............................................................................................................................................................................

...............................................................................................................................................................................

...............................................................................................................................................................................

...............................................................................................................................................................................

...............................................................................................................................................................................

...............................................................................................................................................................................

...............................................................................................................................................................................

# Weekly Meal planner + Journal

|     | BREAKFAST | LUNCH | DINNER | SNACKS |
|-----|-----------|-------|--------|--------|
| MON |           |       |        |        |
| TUE |           |       |        |        |
| WED |           |       |        |        |
| THU |           |       |        |        |
| FRI |           |       |        |        |
| SAT |           |       |        |        |
| SUN |           |       |        |        |

Who can support you in your dietary changes? How will you involve them in your journey?

........................................................................................................................................

........................................................................................................................................

........................................................................................................................................

........................................................................................................................................

........................................................................................................................................

........................................................................................................................................

........................................................................................................................................

# Weekly Meal planner + Journal

|  | BREAKFAST | LUNCH | DINNER | SNACKS |
|---|---|---|---|---|
| MON | | | | |
| TUE | | | | |
| WED | | | | |
| THU | | | | |
| FRI | | | | |
| SAT | | | | |
| SUN | | | | |

How do you plan to navigate eating out or social gatherings while adhering to the diet?

........................................................................................................................................
........................................................................................................................................
........................................................................................................................................
........................................................................................................................................
........................................................................................................................................
........................................................................................................................................
........................................................................................................................................

# Weekly Meal planner + Journal

|  | BREAKFAST | LUNCH | DINNER | SNACKS |
|---|---|---|---|---|
| MON | | | | |
| TUE | | | | |
| WED | | | | |
| THU | | | | |
| FRI | | | | |
| SAT | | | | |
| SUN | | | | |

How does your exercise routine complement your dietary changes? What adjustments might you need to make?

..................................................................................................................................................................

..................................................................................................................................................................

..................................................................................................................................................................

..................................................................................................................................................................

..................................................................................................................................................................

..................................................................................................................................................................

..................................................................................................................................................................

# Weekly Meal planner + Journal

|  | BREAKFAST | LUNCH | DINNER | SNACKS |
|---|---|---|---|---|
| MON |  |  |  |  |
| TUE |  |  |  |  |
| WED |  |  |  |  |
| THU |  |  |  |  |
| FRI |  |  |  |  |
| SAT |  |  |  |  |
| SUN |  |  |  |  |

**How will you handle days when you might not be able to stick strictly to the diet? What is your plan for getting back on track?**

...................................................................................................................................................
...................................................................................................................................................
...................................................................................................................................................
...................................................................................................................................................
...................................................................................................................................................
...................................................................................................................................................
...................................................................................................................................................

# Weekly Meal planner + Journal

|  | BREAKFAST | LUNCH | DINNER | SNACKS |
|---|---|---|---|---|
| MON |  |  |  |  |
| TUE |  |  |  |  |
| WED |  |  |  |  |
| THU |  |  |  |  |
| FRI |  |  |  |  |
| SAT |  |  |  |  |
| SUN |  |  |  |  |

**What motivates you to follow this diet? How can you keep that motivation high throughout your journey?**

..................................................................................................................................................................

..................................................................................................................................................................

..................................................................................................................................................................

..................................................................................................................................................................

..................................................................................................................................................................

..................................................................................................................................................................

..................................................................................................................................................................

**Scan the QR code below to get a surprise bonus**

www.ingramcontent.com/pod-product-compliance
Lightning Source LLC
Chambersburg PA
CBHW082235220526
45479CB00005B/1240